The Dancer's Book of Health.

The DANCER'S Book of HEALTH

L. M. VINCENT, M.D.

A DANCE HORIZONS BOOK
Princeton Book Company, Publishers
Princeton, New Jersey

This reprint edition is published by arrangement
with Andrews and McMeel, Kansas City, MO

Reprinted 1988
A Dance Horizons Book
Princeton Book Company, Publishers
POB 57
Pennington, NJ 08534

The highest function of the teacher
is not so much in imparting knowledge
as in stimulating the pupil
in its love and pursuit.
AMIEL

Contents

Acknowledgments

Thanks to a certain group of people, I'm not wound in adhesive, my thumb isn't stuck in a card catalogue drawer, and a stack of typing paper is no longer blank. Working with them came first as a necessity, but has since become a joy.

George Fernandez and Ralph Jackson helped to set me in the right direction. From there, Eric Case and Dick Dalton, librarians at the Clendening Library of the University of Kansas Medical Center, plodded through with me every inch of the way.

Bernice Jackson, Rare Books librarian of the Clendening History of Medicine Library, never ceased to have a smile, a stack of material, and an offhand, "Oh, by the way—here's a little something else I came across—"

Dr. William Hamilton, Dr. Murray Weisenfeld, Robert LeGrande, Dr. Richard Bachrach, and Dr. John Redford gave graciously of their time and expertise to answer all of my questions, including the ones I didn't know enough to ask.

Dr. Howard Eldfelt and Dr. Norman Martin patiently scouted their X-ray files and permitted me to reproduce their finds.

Dale Durfee, William Batson, and Larry Howell generously provided photography and illustration, and Sylvia Vincent performed typing feats under near-impossible deadline demands, for less reward than the Egyptian slaves got for their pyramid job.

Flora Ann Hall, who, in spite of continually being awakened by frantic late night and early morning calls, never quite learned how not to answer the phone.

And finally, the dancers who served as models, consultants, editors, and friends; who supported, encouraged, and indulged me; and who, most of all, believed in this endeavor:

Liz Hard, Susan Hard, Peggy Ply, Laura Ply, Nita Watson, Carol Feiock, Benecia Carmack, Stephanie Freeman, Nicholas Crumm, Carolyn Hoppe, Flora Ann Hall, Michelle Hamlett, Dennis Landsman, Kathy Bartosh Landsman, and Judy Gillespie. Each in his or her own special way made this book possible, and I share it with them.

Introduction

*Give me the facts, but above all, give me
understanding.*

—SOLOMON

The study of medicine has compounded my respect for and
fascination with the human body, but studying ballet has been
most responsible for enriching and intensifying these
feelings—no activity is more capable of hinting at the human
form's nearness to perfection while so cruelly exposing it to its
most subtle flaws. Sixty-one different athletic activities were
recently evaluated by medical researchers according to physical, mental, and environmental demands; ballet ranked second
only to football by the selected criteria, a finding that shouldn't
surprise anyone with firsthand dance experience. Of course,
dancing requires much more than strength, flexibility, and
endurance. Watching a skilled football player in motion may be
aesthetically pleasing, yet that physical expression of beauty is
incidental to the game, not a conscious pursuit. In his performance, the player isn't burdened with keeping the foot
pointed, controlling those last few millimeters of maximum
extension, preserving the proper line, or harder yet, holding a
picture-perfect smile behind the face mask.

Interest in the dance is increasing rapidly in this country:
more than 350 dance companies are registered with the American Association of Dance Companies, and dance audiences
have increased from an estimated one million persons ten years
ago to well over twelve million in 1976. What was once an
almost totally neglected topic in the medical literature—

11

injuries experienced specifically by the dancer—is appearing with greater frequency in all varieties of journals. And considering America's obsession with health and fitness, it seems paradoxical that dancers—who, of all people, have such a sharply developed inherent "feel" for the control and limitations of their bodies and are so dependent on sound health—often have only a vague, if not completely ignorant, conception of their bodily workings. Naturally a dancer's concerns are concrete—a frustrated ballet pupil, grimacing with pain and disgust as she forces more height à la seconde by tugging at the underside of her thigh with her hand, cares only about that leg's stubborn betrayal, not kinesiology. Yet any further understanding or added awareness of that body in a different dimension might serve to make her a healthier, if not a better, dancer.

Bluntly stated, a dancer's health can be as fragile as stale brownies, mainly because what is a relatively minor medical problem for anyone else can have the disastrous dimensions of a *Titanic* or a *Hindenburg* for a dancer. This I state with complete conviction, having learned it the hard way. Roughly two and a half weeks before my first public performance, I experienced the most minor of thigh muscle pulls. My personal response to the injury was at best neurotic, irrational, hysterical, and totally unscientific. I immersed myself in a mummy's worth of bandages, spread on balms like margarine, and submitted my flesh to heat, cold, Saran Wrap, massage, and everything else imaginable. I hounded the medical librarians for every pertinent medical text and article, and pestered anyone who even remotely resembled an orthopedist, all the while hobbling like Tiny Tim amidst an odorous cloud of menthol and camphor. It was a case of one who had frequently prescribed "tincture of time" for "insignificant" miseries being on the other side of the medical fence. Mind you, all of this hullabaloo was over a role that with some exaggeration and flattery might be called a walk-on and an injury that was without doubt the most miniscule ever sustained by any dancer in the history of the world (although this cannot be documented). Miraculously my thigh healed and I did my bit, but more importantly I was beginning to relate to the psyche of a dancer. No longer did I wonder why dancers are generally such suckers as regards fads, fallacies, and quackery. But who could draw the line between hocus-pocus health myths and plausibly effective practices, bizarre or not, that evolved from experience, superstition, common sense, or ignorance? Shamefully I admitted to being completely baffled (I wasn't even sure how heating balms worked) and realized that dancers have much to learn from medicine, but something special to offer as well. So, partially out of guilt, but mainly out of curiosity, I temporarily pushed aside my balms, heat pads, ace wraps, and adhesive tape and decided to write this book—less with the perspective of a doctor than that of a lover of the dance.

Since the endeavor has left me still baffled, though to a lesser degree, I offer a remark from Oscar Wilde as a literary rationalization: "Truth is never pure and rarely simple." As a further defense, I hide behind the skirts of the hackneyed medical axiom: "Medicine is not an exact science." Any attempt at the pretense of expounding the right way to deal with dance problems would be going out on a limb longer than a bad version of Swan Lake. Fortunately I have no such pretensions.

This book is not specifically intended to be a first-aid handbook, a textbook on dance-related injuries and problems, or in any way a substitute for proper medical evaluation and care. Although it generally concerns itself with "dancing" and "health," there has been no attempt at comprehensiveness. Many topics have been glossed over or neglected—therapeutic exercise, taping techniques, the problems of the young dancer, and the upper extremities, just for starters. The omission of these topics is not intended to undermine their importance; rather, it reflects my own personal interests and intent. In the true spirit of eclecticism, this book is a potpourri of many different things: some basic concepts, hard and soft facts, useful and useless information, suggestions and tidbits, digressions, trivia, authorial self-indulgence, and occasional nonsense. In my perusal of dance literature—both medical and nonmedical—I have always found something to be lacking; I hope that this book can satisfy the need for a very practical, impractical book for dancers.

Maybe a dancer who reads this book might be spared some needless anxiety over a trivial injury that at first appears devastating. Maybe he or she can avert a more serious or chronic problem by seeking proper attention for what appears to be a simple nuisance. Or maybe a dancer might find a single tidbit contained herein useful or fun. Regardless, if this book can help to acquaint the dancer with another aspect of his or her body, or if it can aid in the acquisition of a different kind of "feel" for a body that is capable of such divine expression and profound beauty, then the effort will have been well worthwhile.

PART ONE

Making Connections

1

The Body and Injury

. . . none of us is perfect. I, for myself,
am peculiarly susceptible to draughts.
—OSCAR WILDE

Man's musculoskeletal and nervous systems are estimated to be the product of perhaps 350 million years of evolution. Whatever the determining factors might have been, one thing is for certain: natural selection had no concern for the development of a better ballet dancer. The Neanderthals obviously didn't fall out of earthly favor because their turn-out wasn't as good as Cro-Magnon's, and humans, unlike horses, are not constructed for walking on their toes. Possibly even the transition to the upright posture from all fours was a shade too ambitious, considering all the people walking around with low back pain.* The point merely being that classical ballet imposes physical demands that our bodies are not necessarily suited for, either anatomically or physiologically. Are you flashing back to a stern ballet mistress slamming her cane to the rhythm of "ALL . . . INJURIES . . . ARE THE RESULT . . . OF BAD . . . TRAINING"? The sentiment of that familiar premise is quite touching, but its validity is superseded by naive romanticism. Granted, incorrect technique and bad

---

* This complicated medical, legal, and philosophical question is fortunately beyond the scope of this book.

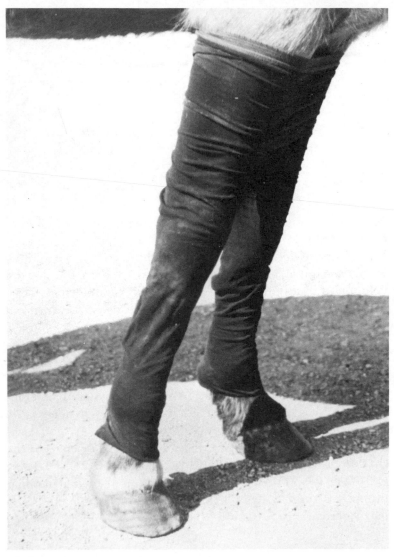

Perfect legs and feet for pointe work, but poor turnout.
Photo by Jan Vincent

training are responsible for more than their fair share of problems, but the fact remains that the human machine is not a dancing machine, and nothing serves better than dancing to prove the point. Nor can we neglect the accident—"an inevitable occurrence due to the action of immutable natural laws," according to Ambrose Bierce. What's going to prevent a mythical dancing machine from executing series of chaînés into the path of a falling set, the grand battement of a myopic corps member, or a banana peel, for that matter?

Aside from the usual lackluster aches, pains, and miseries, the majority of dance injuries fall into two basic categories: those due to accidents, and those which fall under the wastebasket heading of "overuse syndrome." The latter come about with continual stresses (bad technique contributes to many), when any weak bodily link may rear its ugly head with maladies such as shin splints, bursitis, or chronic tendinitis. According to the orthopedist for the New York City Ballet, an average of fifteen to twenty dancers out of ninety will be sidelined for any given performance. According to workmen's compensation claims of a large professional ballet company for 1976, each company member had roughly an 80 percent chance of missing some time from work due to occupational injury. Not surprisingly, about half of the complaints were from the ankle down, but by no means were difficulties with the neck, back, hip, or knees excluded from the motley listing of ailments.

Dance-related injuries follow predictable patterns and are dependent on many variables besides the three most obvious: the basic raw materials with which a dancer must, of necessity, work; technical competence; and dancing conditions. Males logically have a different pattern of difficulties from females: spared many of the foot problems that are related to pointe work, they are more inclined towards ankle and back vulnerability because of the emphasis on jumping, leaping, and partnering. The style of dance and the biases of the choreographer will similarly dictate the types of stresses and strains. The aspiring dancer under sixteen, still growing, has an entirely different set of problems from her more mature counterpart. Time of life is not the sole temporal factor: injuries characteristically are most prevalent in the late afternoon before a season's opening, reflecting the fatigue of increased work schedules and building psychological tensions and pressures. The end of a long, tiring tour is also often heralded by a rapid rise in the injury rate.

The demands of dance provide their own weeding out process, à la Darwin. A pigeon-toed adolescent is never going to become a prima ballerina, no matter what. Paraprofessionals and dilettantes may successfully avoid the grueling selection process, only to get into trouble by trying to do more than they are able, forcing what just isn't there. Whatever our aspirations in dance may be—fun, profit, conditioning, or the only way there is—all of us ultimately confront our limitations at our relatively different levels.

2

Bits and Pieces

There is more wisdom in your body
than in your deepest philosophy.
—FRIEDRICH NIETZSCHE, *Human, All Too Human*

A ballerina is holding a high arabesque sur la pointe, and as we watch, perhaps unconsciously holding our breaths, we aren't giving much thought to bones and muscles and such. Let's digress and leave her balanced, for the moment, and consider some of those bits and pieces.

BONES

Usually we tend to think of bones as those of a dried up display skeleton, completely static and serving only as a framework or protective structure for the rest of the body. Granted, bony architecture is the basic determinant of possible ranges of motion, and although it can't be changed in a large sense, it does alter dramatically in the microscopic sense. Bone is a living dynamic tissue which is constantly being remodeled throughout life; it functions as the organ responsible for the production of red blood cells, and as a storage house for calcium, phosphorus, and other minerals. The continual deposition and reabsorption of bone (with a positive balance of deposition in youth and a negative one with the advent of age) comes

21

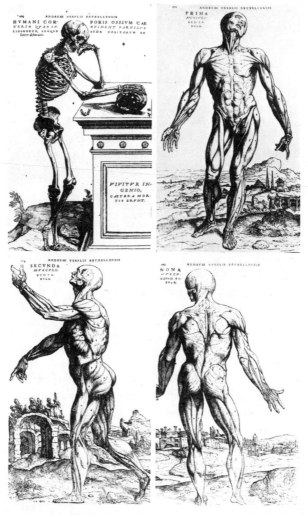

Just for a look under the skin, these reproductions are taken from the first edition (1543) of *De humani corporis fabrica librorum epitome,* by Andreas Vesalius (it isn't in paperback). These fine woodcuts, the first examples of human anatomy ever to be depicted, are commonly attributed to Jan Stephan van Calcar. —COURTESY OF THE LOGAN CLENDENING HISTORY OF MEDICINE LIBRARY, UNIVERSITY OF KANSAS MEDICAL CENTER

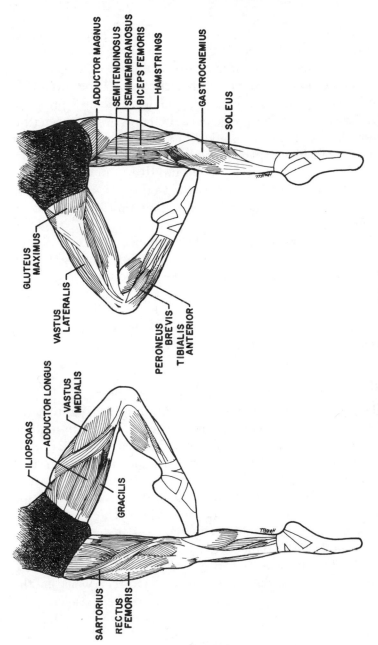

Superficial musculature of the leg.

about in response to cell death, factors causing the removal of calcium and of other minerals, and—of most concern to the dancer—because of stress. Disuse or withdrawal of mechanical stress results in a degenerative process of bone known as disuse osteoporosis. Similarly, there is laying down of more new bone in areas where greater mechanical demands are imposed (this remodeling of bone in relation to stress is known as Wolf's Law). All of which explains why a bony spur can develop in an area subjected to repeated friction and stress, and why the first toe joint underlying a bunion reacts to the excess pressure by enlarging. More subtle is the fact that there appear to be certain bony developmental changes that are unique to classical ballet dancers. A good number of dancers who have done pointe work for many years may have a slightly increased width and altered shape of the long leg bones and several metatarsals. This is an insignificant alteration that is the result of a normal body reaction, but I find it intriguing that sometimes X-rays of the legs and feet alone might be enough basis for saying: "She dances."

JOINTS

The articulations of bones may be immovable, slightly movable, or freely movable. For anyone concerned with motion, the latter type—the so-called diarthrodial joint—naturally holds the most interest. Diarthrodial joints are characterized by a fluid-filled joint cavity and a tough fibrous capsule which completely encloses the joint; lining the cavity is the thin fluid-secreting membrane called synovium. The thick and viscous synovial fluid resembles the white of an egg; its job is to nourish and lubricate the cartilage that covers the bone articulations. The cartilage itself is a smooth, bluish-white surface covering that absorbs shock, prevents direct wear on the bones, and alters the fit of the joint (in some joints the cartilage is more specialized and is given a special name, such as the meniscus of the knee). Normally there is only a slight amount of this lubricating substance overlying the cartilage, but injuries involving joints can sometimes cause profuse secretion and even evident swelling.

LIGAMENTS

Bones are held together by ligaments (from the Latin *ligare*, to bind or tie); these tough and practically nonelastic bands of tissue may blend in with and reinforce the fibrous joint capsule, join the bone ends together within the capsule, or may not be closely associated with the joint capsule at all. Ligaments maintain joint stability and limit range of motion, but they don't act alone in these regards. Fit of the joint and surrounding musculature are also factors in stabilization; similarly, limitation of movement may be a reflection of muscle length or anatomical structure (impingement of bone against bone is going to stop motion no matter how stretched out the soft tissues are).

Which brings us to flexibility, the capacity to yield to passive strength and to relax, and thereby demonstrate a large range of motion. Flexibility depends upon the stretch of soft tissues, particularly ligaments and muscles. Muscle tissue is elastic and must not be considered analogous to the relatively nonelastic ligaments. An unduly stretched ligament cannot return to its original length, and there is no evidence that ligament strength, like muscle strength, can be increased by exercise. Ligament laxity may permit good flexibility and extension, but without adequate muscular strength, this can be at the expense of stability and support, with the dancer compounding her vulnerability to injury.

BURSAE

Anywhere that soft structures in the body are submitted to a frictional rubbing, friction is reduced by bursae, closed fibrous sacs lined by a synovial membrane. As a by-product of dancing's repetitive movements and extremes of motion, bursae get a good workout. There may be as many as eleven different bursae in the vicinity of the knee joint alone; we remain totally unappreciative and ignore these friction-proofers until we become acutely aware of their presence by their inflammation from too much work, a condition known as bursitis.

MUSCLES

The individual muscle fibers that make up muscles are unable to increase in number; they can only change in dimension. This principle is unsubtly illustrated by the muscular enlargement, or hypertrophy, of weight lifters, who achieve tremendous bulk with certain types of training. Conversely, with disuse muscle cells shrink in size or undergo atrophy (for the dancer this may be brought about by the immobilization necessitated by an injury). What the muscle cells lack in ability to multiply, they make up for by their knack for contracting. With contraction, a muscle can shorten up to about fifty percent of its original length, or it can increase its tension without shortening (the isotonic as compared to isometric contraction). In the simplest terms, by voluntarily contracting a skeletal muscle that crosses over a joint—a muscle originating from a fixed point on one bone and inserting, usually by a tendon*, onto

---

* Perhaps you've noticed the similarity between the words "tendon" and "tendu." Both have the same origins from the Greek "to stretch." A tendon is thus the stretched or elongated part of muscle. Tendons join muscle to bone, ligaments join bone to bone.

another—we produce movement.

Muscles never act alone, although most of the credit goes to the so-called prime mover, the chief muscle or chief member of a group of muscles responsible for a particular movement. Accessory muscles that aid in the action may be fixators, which contract isometrically to stabilize the origin of the prime mover so it can work efficiently, or synergists, which either aid in the general movement or stabilize intermediate joints to prevent unwanted movements. Working in opposition are the antagonists, which must relax by reflex action before the contraction can take place to begin with. As an example, take a développé en avant. The prime mover for the straightening at the knee is the powerful quadriceps group; the stretch, however, is at the back of the leg, in the antagonistic hamstrings. On the other hand, when the knee is bent or flexed, the quadriceps will be subserviently stretched in opposition to the contracting hamstrings. Similarly, the adductor muscles, which form the normal contour of the inner thigh, must relax and stretch when the abductors are employed to lift the leg to the side.

To briefly clarify some terms: *abduction* refers to the movement of a body part away from the midline; the opposite movement is *adduction*. *Rotation* implies the pivoting of a bone on its axis, and may be either *internal*—toward the body midline—or *external*—away from the body midline (en dedans and en dehors, if you will). Thus turn-out is known in scientific circles (if it ever comes up) as "external rotation of the hips." Bending or folding movements are called *flexion*, while *extension* is the straightening of a body part or a return from flexion. Dancers commonly speak of "extension" in the loose sense of overall flexibility—for a dancer who achieves considerable height doing a battement en avant, her so-called good extension is actually (anatomically speaking, anyway) good flexion at the hips. For most descriptive purposes, it's probably easier to use ballet terminology, as dance movements almost always involve combinations of these rigid definitions, especially since nearly every motion includes some degree of hip "external rotation."

Different varieties of movement require a differing interplay of antagonistic and synergistic muscles. With a rapid and powerful movement (such as grand battement), there is unresisted shortening by the prime mover with the antagonist completely relaxed. In slower, more controlled movements, the body part moves in the direction of the muscles exerting the strongest pull, and there is continual readjustment of tension in the antagonists. The reciprocating action of antagonists and synergists increases the steadiness and accuracy of movement—the more accuracy and grace, the greater number of involved muscles. Maintaining balance requires the continuous contraction of antagonistic muscles for fixation; since the synchronous nature of the volleys of nerve impulses stimulating these muscles produces an unsteady muscle response, it is virtually impossible to hold the body completely still in such a position.

So, back to the dancer holding her arabesque. By now her tremor is quite evident, and she conceals the struggle to keep her placement and balance. Perspiration is causing her mascara to run and smear down the side of her eye. She smiles, though, her jaw muscles as tight as a clenched bear trap, manages another half-inch or so of height, and goes on. We, as if having worked hard, breathe a sigh of relief.

INFLAMMATION

> *The human body is the only machine*
> *for which there are no spare parts.*
> —HERMANN M. BIGGS (1859–1923)

No discussion of injury is possible without some—albeit oversimplified—consideration of what goes on under the skin. The body's basic response to damage is an elegantly choreographed cleaning up operation called "inflammation"; its four cardinal manifestations—tumor (swelling), rubor (redness), calor (hotness), and dolor (pain)—were enumerated back in the first century by a physician named Celsus. Most nonmedical people have a very limited and inaccurate concept of this process—they can relate to the "inflamed appendix," "inflamed tonsils," or the "inflammation" of an ingrown toenail or minor scratch, but somehow, the word isn't associated with a muscle pull or an ankle sprain or a bruise.

With any injury, the body tissues—including a myriad of tiny vessels—are damaged, resulting in a mess of spilled blood and other debris. The first step in the sequence of the inflammatory process is an increase in blood flow to the injured area, as well as a greater "leakiness" of the supplying blood vessels. Along with the spillage from the initial insult itself, this accounts for swelling which, visible to the naked eye or not, accompanies all injuries. This response also permits better accessibility for the corps of white cells, antibacterial proteins, and other substances that gather on the scene. The accumulating white cells are of different types and have different jobs; some specialize in swallowing and killing any intruding bacteria (polymorphonuclear leukocytes), while others (macrophages, literally "big eaters") set about consuming other extraneous debris, including many of their cohorts that succumb in the line of duty. During all this excitement, clotting factors are also leaking from the vessels, producing clots to stop the bleeding and setting the stage for resolution.

While the mopping up is underway, specialized cells called fibroblasts are migrating to the injury site and beginning the process of "repair" by forming connective tissue—the soft, tough tissue that is designed for mechanically holding us together, filling the spaces and gaps around all the other tissues of the body. Unlike the lucky lizard, which can regrow a lost tail (bones and all), humans must be content to settle with an end product that is not the original matter, but rather a fibrous scar of a size and extent proportional to the damage. This patchwork has served man admirably, but does have shortcomings for the dancer. Since all-purpose scar tissue does not have the elasticity of muscle, a large enough scar can be a source of tightness and can predispose adjacent areas to injury.

WARMING UP

No dancer needs convincing about the importance of a good warm-up. Preliminary conditioning and flexibility exercises promote performance, adapt the body physiologically to the impending activity, and help to prevent injury. Although actual hard data concerning warm-up in the trained athlete is generally lacking, except for that obtained under extremely artificial conditions, we can easily rationalize why the warm-up is so valuable. First of all, warming up causes an increase in body temperature and metabolism, as well as an augmentation of the rate and volume of blood circulation. Respiratory capacity is increased, not only because oxygen-bounded hemoglobin is more readily at hand, but also because the hemoglobin surrenders its oxygen less reluctantly to the tissues (additionally, oxygen stored in muscle is more readily relinquished at higher temperatures). Nerve impulses travel faster in warm muscle and muscle viscosity is less, making contraction easier and more efficient. The optimum temperature for the speed of chemical reactions and metabolism involved in muscle functioning is in the neighborhood of 102 to 103 degrees Fahrenheit, and the only efficient way to reach this temperature in the muscle is working the muscle.

A thorough warm-up includes general preliminary exercises and stretches followed by more specific movements, steps, and combinations, initiated gradually and vigorous enough to cause perspiration. Passive means for warming up, such as hot showers or massage, are not satisfactory; and although leg and body warmers may be of some value in retaining body warmth (especially in cold rehearsal rooms or draughty backstage areas), it must be kept in mind that they are only a superficial aid, an inadequate substitute for body heat generated by muscular activity. The muscles most frequently pulled during activity that has not been preceded by a sufficient warm-up are the antagonists to the strong contracting muscles. "Cold" hamstrings will relax or lengthen slowly and incompletely when called to do so by contraction of the quadriceps for a développé. This lack of synergistic muscular coordination can retard efficient and correct movement and cause tearing of the hamstring muscle fibers.

Ballistic forms of stretching (bobbing, lunging, bouncing) can result in muscle or tendon injuries and should be avoided. Most dancers learn early on (or should, anyway) that a more satisfactory way to stretch the hamstrings than plopping the fingers to the floor by a jerking drop from the waist is to bend at the knees, place the fingers or palms on the ground, and slowly straighten up. The controlled stretch will inherently prevent injury by taking advantage of a spinal reflex known as the myotatic reflex. When a critical level of tension builds up in an antagonistic muscle that is undergoing stretch, the muscle will automatically be triggered to contract, thus avoiding overstretch. Additionally, controlled movement allows pain to signal the build-up of excessive amounts of tension on a muscle before something gives and it's too late.

3

Hurts and Bumps

*The chapter of accidents
is the longest chapter in the book.*
—JOHN WILKES (1727–1797)

Strains, sprains, and contusions account for a goodly percentage of the problems that a dancer will inevitably encounter at some point in his or her career. The precipitating traumatic incident will be accompanied by immediate pain and a certain degree of bleeding in the tissues. The amount of swelling which develops does not necessarily indicate the severity of the injury. For example, rapid and extensive swelling may simply be due to the involvement of a local vein in what is a minor overall injury; on the other hand, it might signify extensive tissue damage. Determing the type and severity of the injury is the job of the physician; in his evaluation he will use the criteria of pain, spasm, functional loss, and instability. What the dancer should do first is recognize that the pain is the body's way of saying "stop dancing." The second step is to immediately minimize the initial injury response by application of cold, compression, and elevation. Since blood accumulation in the tissues must be completely absorbed before the area is back to normal, controlling the amount of hemorrhage and swelling by these simple first-aid measures can have a profound effect on the extent and length of resultant disability. If you have even the slightest feeling you may have injured yourself, play it safe and get the ice right away—it can't hurt and it's well worth the slight inconvenience if it can prevent a swollen leg a couple of hours later. Remember this above all: *Initial heat application will only increase the amount of bleeding and swelling and has absolutely no place in the treatment of an acute injury.*

STRAINS

Excessive stretching of a muscle can cause tearing of the muscle fibers anywhere along the muscle-tendon unit. This is the common "muscle pull," and it may range in severity from a mild pull (first-degree strain), in which only a small number of fibers is involved with no appreciable bleeding; to a moderate pull (second-degree strain), in which more fibers are damaged but the muscle-tendon unit is still intact; to a severe pull (third-degree strain), in which there is complete rupture—either muscle from muscle, muscle from tendon, or tendon from bone. In the case of a minor pull, treatment with cold for the first twenty-four to forty-eight hours followed by heat application for symptomatic relief along with rest for a short period may be adequate; a severe pull, on the other hand, usually requires open surgical repair and total rehabilitation.

So much for textbook theory. Fortunately, the majority of muscle pulls sustained by dancers are relatively minor, but many dancers get into trouble even with these injuries because of failure to give them the proper care and respect. A hopeful "I think I can work it out" may, for the dancer, become famous last words. A muscle pull cannot, repeat, *cannot*, be "worked out" or "run out." Any attempt to prematurely push such an injury inevitably leads to greater tearing of muscle fibers and an increase in scarring. Remember that scar tissue is inelastic and has a tendency toward tightness; too much stretch before elasticity is adequately restored to the area can easily cause re-injury. Further negligence results in a downhill spiral, with what should have been a soon-healed minor disability even-tuating in a chronic aggravation. To avoid this hassle, first and foremost, allow the muscle time to heal, and second, go easy and don't push when returning to dancing. Restore elasticity to the area by gentle stretching, and be more concerned with how often you stretch rather than how hard.

SPRAINS

Sprains involve ligaments and are the result of direct or indirect trauma to a joint, characteristically caused by a sudden twisting injury. The amount of pain, swelling, and disability—as with strains—is dependent upon the extent of the damage. Sprains are also categorized from mild (first-degree), involving a minor tearing of ligament fibers, to severe (third-degree), which is the complete tearing of a ligament. The forces causing a sprain may also disrupt the synovial lining of the joint and produce hemorrhage in the joint itself (hemarthrosis). Severe sprains can result in cartilage damage as well as bone fractures.

In addition to the immediate application of cold, compres-sion, and elevation, immobilization is also exceedingly impor-tant, because in a significant sprain the ligamentous support may be quite compromised and hence vulnerable to more tearing. Further treatment depends upon the recommenda-tions of a physician and will usually include (after twenty-four to forty-eight hours) the use of heat or contrast baths, further avoidance of joint stress, and, as soon as medically indicated, a physical therapy rehabilitative regimen, typically beginning with range of motion and progressing to weight-bearing exer-cise, and possibly including massage or other physical therapy modalities if advisable or accessible. Sprains are common injuries in dancers and are often difficult to evaluate. For example, on the outside of the ankle there are three ligaments; an ankle sprain in this region can involve one, two, or all three. Accurate assessment, particularly with swelling complicating the picture, is no mean trick. A severe sprain could require placing the dancer in plaster, and although an experienced orthopedic surgeon will make a maximum effort not to use a cast if it isn't absolutely necessary, he realizes that it can be disastrous to let a ligament heal loosely. If indicated, adequate immobilization is of much higher priority than the avoidance of some resultant muscle atrophy, because once a ligament has become loose or chronically stretched, no amount of exercise can restore direct stability to the joint.

CONTUSIONS (BRUISES)

Contusions or bruises arise from a direct blow to any part of the dancer's body, with bleeding into the tissues from the insult resulting in the all-to-familiar discoloration and pain. The amount of reaction depends on the body part involved; a blow to the calf won't produce a shiner as a similar smack to the face would, for example. Unfortunately for the dancer, the foot and shin, which are the most vulnerable, are fairly sensitive.

Contusions are likewise categorized from first to third degree, but most bruises encountered generally won't put the dancer out of commission. An important exception is, of course, the stone bruise, a contusion on the bottom of the foot which results from hard repetitive pounding on the floor. Immediate application of cold and compression followed by a gradual stretch to relieve muscle spasm (responsible for most of the discomfort in minor contusions) can help alleviate some of the discoloration and discomfort.* The normal bruise will rarely become worse after the first twenty-four hours or so, but heat application may be useful in some cases after this length of time, when the hemorrhaging will have long since ceased. With an unsightly bruise that shows through light-colored tights for a performance, my only medical suggestion is the application of clown white, pancake base, and/or powder (all available without prescription).

---

* As a sidelight, it's interesting to note that Thomas Sydenham, a seventeenth-century physician, advised young fledgling doctors to read *Don Quixote de la Mancha* as a practical guide for good medical management. One recalls that the Don, although he did not dance, was continually getting bashed about, and Sancho Panza was forever concocting home remedies for plasters, poultices, and balms. A particular remedy for contusions consisted of oil, wine, salt, and rosemary, and although in my experience this has absolutely no effect whatsoever, it does make a fairly good salad dressing.

4

Soaks and Strokes

*Now King David was old and stricken in years; and
they covered him with clothes, but he could get no
heat. Wherefore his servants said unto him: Let
there be sought for my Lord the King a young
virgin; and let her stand before the King, and be a
companion unto him; and let her lie in thy bosom,
that my Lord the King may get heat.*
—THE BIBLE, 1 Kings 1:1–2

HEAT

Let no one wonder how people got by before the invention
of the whirlpool. Since ancient times, heat has been employed
as a form of treatment, not only from the use of blankets or
sweat baths, but, as the above quotation indicates, from the
vigorous warmth of youth (this therapeutic application of vir-
gins was highly recommended up through the seventeenth
century). All dancers employ therapeutic heat, if only to exploit
the relaxing effects of being in a hot tub after an exhausting day.
Oddly enough, no one is exactly sure of the mechanism behind
heat's relief of pain and muscular tension, but other beneficial
effects are more clearly understood. A temperature rise in an
area of injury brings about an increase in local metabolism and a
dilation of the blood vessels. More blood flow insures a greater
supply of oxygen and nutrients to the surrounding tissues,
permitting a faster clearing of waste products, and expediting

37

the arrival on the scene of the cells involved in the healing process. Thus, heat has the dual capacity of providing symptomatic relief of pain as well as facilitating the body's natural healing processes.

As a general unwritten and unproven medical law, moist heat works better than dry heat. To obtain this effect when the luxury of a tub isn't available or practical, place a hot, wet washcloth on the area of misery, cover securely with Saran Wrap and a towel, and then use a regular heating pad. Since it's fairly difficult to dance while using a heat pad, Saran Wrap is rapidly becoming an indispensable first-aid item for the dancer. Wrapping a sore limb with a layer or two of Saran retains the natural body warmth and perspiration: a pretty sneaky and easy way of getting fairly constant moist heat. This is particularly useful for those with chronic tendon problems. One can recycle plastic cleaner's bags or sandwich bags by snipping off the closed end for the toes and slipping over the foot under the tights to keep the ankle warm. Unfortunately, plastic and Saran may shine through the tights under performance lights, so the heat must come off when the show goes on. Although one physician I've encountered believes this practice can overheat and exhaust the muscles, the general consensus among most physicians is favorable, and most Saran-Wrapped dancers will swear by it. Always wrap without tension, and, to be judicious, don't remain bagged for more than overnight or a few hours at a time.

Overzealous use of external heating sources can inadvertently lead to burning. Since stinging pain may or may not accompany the burning process, it is best to limit the treatment to twenty-to-thirty-minute intervals, repeated three to four times throughout the day. If the temperature is within the usual therapeutic range (110–115 degrees Fahrenheit), the desired effect should be obtained within this length of time.

Whenever using a heating pad, remember that it is easier to be burned lying on the pad rather than under it, since the weight of the body reduces blood flow through the skin, hindering adequate removal of excessive heat by blood flow to other, cooler parts of the body.

Steam Baths and Saunas. Steam baths and saunas are currently out of the medical vogue. Many people contend that they are of questionable value, that they do little more than stimulate sweating and produce widespread dilation of the blood vessels, an effect which can sometimes lead to a drastic lowering of blood pressure and can even be deadly for old or physically unfit people. Although a sense of mild fatigue and complete relaxation occurs in many who take a steam bath or sauna, a hot bath or a massage can probably be just as effective for winding down. If you choose to indulge, don't overdo.

Heating Balms. For those who have always wondered how balms and ointments work, wonder no more. Preparations such as Ben-Gay, Heet, Absorbine, and Sloan's are called rubefacients (literally, to make red) and are all irritants to the skin. The local irritation produces dilation of the small blood vessels near the surface of the skin, hence an increase in circulation and warmth. The most common ingredients used as irritants in these commercial remedies include methyl salicylate (oil of wintergreen), menthol, camphor, thymol, and eucalyptol. If using these products, avoid also using heating pads or lamps, as the skin may burn or blister (this doesn't appear to be the case with Saran Wrap, which works well in combination with balms). Also avoid contact with the eyes by carefully washing the residue from your hands.

Deep Heating. Both radiant heat (that from a heat lamp) and conductive heat (that directly applied in such forms as hot water or pads) are relatively superficial, with maximum temperature increases occurring in the skin and progressively less heat farther down (there doesn't appear to be any significant temperature rise beyond one to two centimeters below the skin). Thus, despite any sedative or psychological relief, direct effects on deeply injured tissue are negligible or nonexistent. Conversive heating (also called deep heating or medical diathermy) is achieved by forms of physical energy penetrating the skin and being transformed into heat deep in the tissues. The three types of energy in use at the present time include shortwave (high-frequency current), microwave (energy in the form of electromagnetic waves), and ultrasound (energy consisting of mechanical vibrations). Diathermy is entirely under the domain of the medical specialist, and all machines are operated under regulations established by the Federal Communications Commission.

The particular modality selected for therapy depends upon the type of injury, the amount of tissue involved, and the location. Ultrasound seems to be particularly useful in the loosening of adhesions; it is claimed that pain which persists following sprains can also be relieved by this method, which may accelerate the healing of the injury. Unfortunately, this is currently a gray area, and it is difficult to adequately assess the overall value of these techniques for the dancer's particular problems.

COLD

For the most part, cold produces the opposite effects of heat: a decrease in temperature, a lowering of metabolic activity, and vascular constriction with a decrease in blood flow. Thus, the prompt application of cold is the treatment of choice to minimize the swelling and hemorrhage that are the initial results of injury. In addition, cold has a numbing effect that greatly reduces pain. Application is most convenient by ice packs or cold-water baths (cold running water seems to cause less numbing achiness than ice) at five-minute intervals for about the first thirty minutes.

Heat has been the traditional mode of treatment in the later stages of injury; that is, after twenty-four to forty-eight hours, when all bleeding in the tissues has subsided. However, another effect of cold is the reduction of muscle spasm, which allows active or passive exercise that is helpful in preventing muscle atrophy and diminishing adhesions. For this reason, some physicians may recommend the continued use of cold, depending on their own experience, personal biases, the type of injury, and the patient's previous health history. Generally this will consist of ice massage for ten minutes (or soaking in cold water up to twenty minutes), followed by brief bouts of the appropriate exercises. Other physicians show a preference for alternating hot and cold soaks, or contrast baths, for certain types of injuries, particularly ankle sprains. If recommended, the procedure for this method is hot-water (108–110 degrees Fahrenheit) immersion for approximately four minutes, followed by cold-water immersion (36–40 degrees Fahrenheit) for about a minute, continued for twenty to thirty minutes, three to four times a day.

Understanding the physiological effects of heat and cold, consider the situation: a dancer has a minor mishap on a slick floor, grimaces a bit, and continues to hobble through rehearsal. Fellow dancers express their concern and then promptly offer their own extra stockings and warm-ups. The injured dancer accepts these graciously, wraps up the aching part, and naively says, "Thanks, I'll keep it real warm and it will be all right." Obviously this practice is totally erroneous and very possibly detrimental: if the injury is such that there is significant bleeding in the tissues, the dancer could remove the warming garments later only to find a foot or ankle having the proportions of Popeye's forearms (after spinach therapy). Dancers often have to deal with swollen feet, particularly if performing requires them to go from pointe shoes to character shoes, and back again into pointe shoes. Cold running water can perform miracles for this dilemma: nothing more than a sink, adequate plumbing, and a few minutes is needed to get the feet back into the shoes. A desperate dancer may even resort to placing her feet in the toilet bowl and flushing for an instant, swelling-reducing whirlpool—a known fact which I put forth with an almost-straight face and no additional comment.

MASSAGE

> Boy, after all these classes and rehearsals I
> ache all over. What I really need is a good
> tripsisparaskeulasthke.
> –Hypothetical statement by a dancer,
> circa A.D. 150

Massage has been known by many names throughout its long history as one of the oldest forms of therapeutic measures known to medicine.* The Chinese described forms of massage in cases dating back almost three thousand years; they, as well as the ancient Egyptians, Greeks, and Romans, attributed great importance to it. Although its popularity has waned in more recent times, since World War II its value and effectiveness in treatment have become more appreciated.

Appropriately performed massage produces effects on the nervous and muscular systems and on the local and general

---

* Known simply as anointing or rubbing in the Homeric Age (100 B.C.); Hippocrates called it *Anatripsis* (460–380 B.C.); Galen called it *Apotherapeia* or *Tripsisparaskeulasthke* (A.D. 130–200); and Toga Islanders used either *Toogi-Toogi, Mili,* or *Fota.*

circulation of the blood and lymph. Proper administration may be useful for relief of pain and swelling, relaxation of muscle tension, and stretching of adhesions; overall, it may help maintain the muscles in the best possible state of nutrition, flexibility, and vitality, so that after recovery from injury the muscle can function at its maximum. The desired effects are dependent upon the choice of massage movements, as well as the skill of the massage therapist in regulating the duration, quality, intensity, and rhythm of the manipulation. Dancers widely employ massage for general muscle tightness and soreness and for its soothing psychological effects. However, in the case of injuries, massage should only be used with the advice or approval of a medical physician, since its use may be harmful and is definitely contraindicated for the treatment of certain conditions.

Always seek out a licensed massage or physical therapist, preferably one experienced in the treatment of dancers or athletes, and don't be hesitant to shop around, as different therapists may favor different techniques and may vary the intensity with which the techniques are employed. A physician who has had experience in working with dancers recognizes the advantages of working in conjunction with a skilled massage therapist, who may not only aid considerably in rehabilitation, but may also, through knowledgeable and intimate firsthand contact with the soft tissues, be the first to notice other problems or conditions that might require further evaluation by the physician.

PART TWO

Miseries and Coping

5

Pain and Noise

MUSCLE SORENESS

Stop to think about the aches and pains that accompany dancing, and you will recall that there are actually two different types of muscle soreness: that which occurs during or immediately after activity, and the more insidious kind that creeps up hours later. The two types of soreness are recognized as distinct entities, but their exact causes are not completely understood. It is probable that the pain that occurs during or immediately after strenuous exercise is a result of the accumulation of the waste product lactic acid, which irritates the pain receptors in the muscle. This type of pain quickly passes when the exercise ceases, presumably because the lactic acid build-up then has the chance to diffuse from the muscles to the bloodstream.

The reasons for soreness to develop twelve to forty-eight hours after activity and often persist for days are a bit more difficult to pinpoint. Although possible explanations again include excess accumulation of waste products, or actual rupture of some muscle fibers, recent evidence seems to indicate that soreness may result when extensive "pull" traumatizes muscle fibers and causes them to swell. Another theory for the onset of delayed soreness is spasm in fatigued muscles.

The muscle stiffness that often goes hand in hand with muscle soreness may be the result of fluid collecting in muscles during activity; the swollen muscle is shorter and thicker, and hence more resistant to stretching. That general, dragged-out, stiff-in-the-morning phenomenon is probably due to the natural tendency of fascia to contract during rest and inactivity, especially during the inactivity which follows on the heels of an active phase.

Everyone has his or her own particular method of dealing (or not dealing) with muscle soreness—be it baths, balms, alcohol rubdowns in the evening, or complaining. Hearing the moans and groans at the barre during those first few painful minutes of stretching at the beginning of a Monday class, I can't help but believe that dancers require and even thrive on a certain amount of that aching misery. What better evidence is there for having worked hard (the old "if-it-doesn't-hurt-then-you're-not-doing-it-right" philosophy)? And oddly enough, the revolt of that disobedient protoplasm often seems to provide the inspiration and impetus to inflict more torture. After all, no one said it would be easy.

Obviously there is no need to go out and look for any more misery than that which is part and parcel of the occupation, and sensible practices that will decrease the likelihood of soreness will also help to prevent injury. This includes not only a good warm-up and stretch (muscle soreness appears earlier without warm-up), but also a sufficient warming down, which is particularly of help with immediate soreness, as light work hastens the circulatory removal of the waste products (most teachers surely know better than to end classes abruptly after strenuous and exhausting maneuvers). And most importantly, when resuming activity after a temporary layoff or injury, work back gradually and patiently.

Once the pain is present, cold water or ice application for

about fifteen minutes as well as mild exercise is suggested practice for relief (after a contraction, hold the muscle in a stretched position for a brief period, rather than subjecting it to a barrage of lightning-quick repetitions). Regardless of the causes of muscle soreness, the analgesic effects of heat—in whatever form is preferred—are certainly beneficial. For do-it-your-selfers and penny pinchers who fancy balms, make your own muscle rub by stirring ¼ cup mineral oil into a well-mixed concoction containing 1½ cups denatured (type 40) or isopropyl alcohol, ½ cup methyl salicylate, ⅛ teaspoon camphor, and ⅛ teaspoon menthol. Store in a labeled container marked "Keep out of reach of children."

A final word to those with an exceptionally low tolerance for pain: do everything humanly possible to avoid or treat muscle soreness, then adopt the practice of grunting and grimacing when first stretching at the barre, whether it hurts or not.

MUSCLE CRAMPS

Muscle cramps are uncontrollable and painful muscle spasms, usually in weight-bearing muscles, that can occur during sleep, after intensive exercise, or anywhere in the range in between. The activating factors are not entirely clear, but it is known that some cramps may be brought on by the reduction of body salt through perspiration, while others may be due to insufficient blood flow (overuse with excessive build-up of waste products) or injury. The best way to work out a cramp is to slowly stretch the affected muscle within a normal range of motion while putting firm pressure on it through a gentle kneading action. Thorough warming up as well as adequate salt and water intake are good preventative measures for certain types of cramps.

To clarify (or unclarify) some semantics: the term "charleyhorse" is overwhelmingly understood to refer to cramping. With great horror and dismay I learned, however, that according to the standard nomenclature of the American Medical Association, "charleyhorse" refers specifically to a contusion of the quadriceps muscle. Attempting to find some justification for this definition, I came up empty-handed. The actual origin of the word is indeed nebulous, although it probably first surfaced in the 1880s in baseball slang. Some astute linguistic scholars courageously hypothesize that the first victim may actually have been a lamed horse named . . . . At any rate, it was evidently used in reference to pain and/or stiffness in the arms or legs from overexertion, an application which seems equally as remote from muscle cramps as contusions of the quadriceps (it could just as easily have come to mean ingrown toenail or tension headache).

SHIN SPLINTS

Dancers often complain of "shin splints," pain and discomfort in the middle of the leg, usually just to the inside of the tibia. Typically, it is a dull, deep-seated ache that intensifies after vigorous activity and is not particularly responsive to heat or other physical therapy modalities. Distance runners are characteristically prone to this condition in relation to a change in running surfaces; for dancers the major associations appear to be workouts on a hard, unyielding surface (especially pointe work) or an intensive jumping schedule.

Although the exact cause is not known, involvement of the muscles used to bend the foot upwards—the dorsi-flexors (anterior and posterior tibialis muscles)—is suspected. It is possible that partial separation of these muscles occurs with forceful or excessive use. Some researchers feel that athletes who run with their feet turned out and rolling inwards are more prone to the problem; perhaps, for the dancer at least, sickling or rolling over on pointe might be a contributing cause, if the normal stresses and forces aren't enough.

The best preventative advice is to avoid excessive pointe work and jumping on hard surfaces, correct any flaws in technique that might possibly predispose to the problem, and routinely and thoroughly stretch the foot flexors (any warm-up that uses relevé and demi-plié). Continual application of superficial heat is advisable symptomatic treatment, but shin pain that has not resolved after two to three weeks should always be evaluated by a physician, as shin splints must be differentiated from the much more serious problem of stress fractures.

STRESS (FATIGUE) FRACTURES

Definite fractures are not very common in dancers and are usually well treated when they occur, since the severity of the injury warrants immediate medical attention and proper diagnosis by examination and X-ray is generally obvious. Unfortunately, the most common fracture seen in classical ballet dancers, the stress, or fatigue, fracture, is a notable exception to the rule. Diagnosis must be made from the symptoms alone, since initial X-rays may appear entirely normal; in fact, the appearance of X-ray changes may, paradoxically, coincide with recovery.

Stress fractures are the consequence of accumulated impact and shock without any relationship to a single specific traumatic incident. Most frequently they occur in the middle of the front of the tibia, where there are no muscular attachments, but they may be found anywhere along the bone, as well as in the fibula or the femur. Generally their presence is indicated by pain, aching, and local tenderness in the middle of the shin, found to be confined to the bone when examined by a physi-

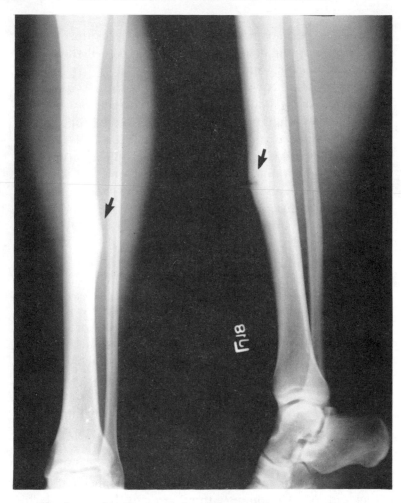

The lower leg X-ray on the right reveals a stress fracture line in the mid-shaft of the tibia (right, arrow). Note the bony thickening in the area of the fracture in another view of the same leg (left, arrow). This bony reaction is part of the normal healing process and may be the only X-ray finding in more subtle stress fractures.

cian. The real danger here is that dancers are apt to identify the condition incorrectly as shin splints; if they then continue dancing, the tibia may break completely and displace.

Proper concern for so-called shin splints can't be overemphasized, and persisting leg pain or aching should always be carefully evaluated. Inadequate shock absorption may be due to faulty technique or fatigue, or a bad dancing floor. Some specialists feel that spongy insoles can reduce impact, but I doubt that shoe inserts are as good a preventative measure as strong feet, a bouncy, yielding surface, and reasonable rehearsal schedules.

If treated early, tibial stress fractures may not require taking a dancer off weight bearing, but *all* dancing must definitely stop. Although the length of rest required depends on the individual case, six weeks is probably the minimum, with abstention for up to three months not unlikely. There is a case in the medical literature of a female dancer who complained of ankle problems as well as of "shin splints." Her ankle was fine, but her legs had had a total of nine stress fractures, requiring her to be in a wheelchair for five months. Finally, need I mention the stupidity of steroid or local anaesthetic injections for shin pain? Masking symptoms can lead to a leg decked out in plaster-cast warmers.

CREAKS AND CLICKS

A classful of dancers warming up with grand plié sounds like a gigantic bowl of Rice Krispies. Most noises are a normal phenomenon, and many dancers just don't feel "right" unless they "free their joints" with a gratifying click. The practice is definitely habit forming and soon becomes an automatic ritual. What causes these strange noises that universally pervade dance studios? Stretching or moving in a certain way can cause a tendon to catch against a bony prominence and then slip over it, creating a snapping sound. This commonly happens at the shoulder, ankle, and hip. In the latter instance, a protruding segment of the femur (greater trochanter) probably catches against the edge of the gluteus maximus muscle.* Deeper clicks may be caused by ligaments of the hip joint (ilio-femoral ligaments) moving over the top of the femur. With bending of the knee, a small bursa may be responsible for the snap as it jumps from one side to the other of the tendon attaching to the kneecap (patellar ligament).

Another mechanism occurs when traction is applied to a joint, especially of the fingers (although I know of no dancer who must crack her knuckles before going onstage, I include this information anyway). X-ray studies have demonstrated that at the moment of the crack, the phalanges spring apart and a gas bubble appears in a joint. Thus, the tension produces a partial vacuum which allows dissolved air to escape (explaining why a knuckle can't be cracked repeatedly; time is needed for the gas to be reabsorbed into the synovial fluid lining the joints). Real world analogies to this mechanism include opening a pop-top can, unstopping a toilet with an old-fashioned plunger, or making a popping sound by flicking the index finger out from inside the cheek. Chances are pretty good that the clicks felt and heard on spinal manipulation come about in the same way.

Noise making is, for the most part, harmless, although in some cases it may be an annoyance or produce slight discomfort. This is probably due to irritation and subsequent swelling

---

* For you do-it-yourselfers who don't already know, the easiest way to click the hip is to lie flat on your back, flex one knee, and pull the bent leg across the body and towards the floor with the opposite arm (internal rotation of the hip).

of the soft tissues caused by constant, repetitive clicking of a joint (usually the hip), in which chronic bursitis may be contributory. In these cases, kicking the habit should be sufficient treatment.

6

Common Nuisances

For chafings caused by footwear,
ash of an old shoe.
—PLINY THE ELDER (A.D. 23–79)

BLISTERS

Pressure and friction on a localized area of skin can result in fluid accumulation between skin layers. Whether the fluid contains blood or is a clear serous material (blood minus the red cells and clotting factors) depends on the depth of tissues involved; in either case, it's a blister and it's a nuisance. Aside from the pain and the possibility of infection, blisters can cause a dancer to compensate for the discomfort and thereby incur other injuries.

Unopened blisters can be protected during activity by a felt or sponge-rubber doughnut applied around the perimeter. On or between the toes, it's easier to use a wisp of lamb's wool, wrapped around the toe without tension and secured by a few winding flicks with the fingers.

A blister ideally should be taken care of by a podiatrist, especially if there are indications of inflammation or irritation. However, as medical assistance may not be readily available or feasible, it is often better to puncture a clear blister before it breaks by itself. Although the procedure is simple, the importance of sterile technique cannot be overemphasized. After thoroughly washing the area with soap and water, prepare the blister area with Merthiolate, iodine, or alcohol. After sterilizing a sharp needle by holding it (preferably by forceps) in a gas flame, insert the needle parallel to the skin close to the edge of the blister, and apply gentle pressure to remove the fluid. The remaining skin layer acts as a protective cover and should be preserved. For about a week afterwards, applying Vaseline and padding (the two sticky sides of adhesive tape stuck together and taped over the area works well) is advisable. Since blood blisters have a greater predisposition to infection, they should not be punctured, but instead should be allowed to reabsorb by themselves.

If a blister inadvertently ruptures, the space between the roof and the skin is already contaminated, and a simple taping of the roof to the underlying skin could seal infection inside the blister. To prevent infection, clean the area with an antiseptic, trim away any loose, ragged edges of the roof that cannot be used for protection, and pack the blister with a salve antiseptic such as zinc oxide. The remaining portion of the roof should be placed over the salve packing and a doughnut or appropriate padding applied. In a couple of days, the old skin can be cut away and the salve removed. If the pain of a blister is incapacitating for performing, application of a topical anaesthetic—Xylocaine (in jelly or ointment form) will temporarily deaden the pain, but antiseptic salve should be reapplied when the performance is over.

The first sign of a blister on the sole of the foot is a reddened and tender area of skin, the so-called hot spot. Prompt application of ice and covering with adhesive tape may keep the actual blister from forming. In addition to careful surveillance for hot spots, unfavorable effects of friction can be minimized by wearing properly fitted shoes and avoiding wrinkles in the tights. Since adhesive tape can sometimes produce friction by sliding

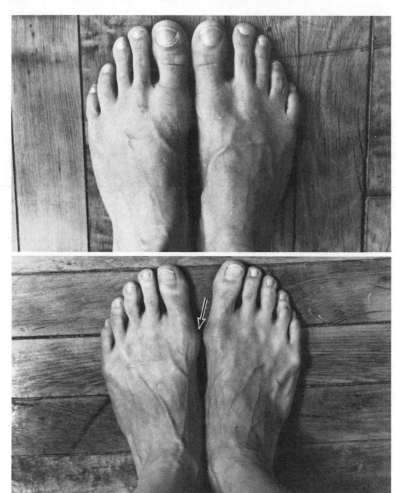

Compare a normal foot (top) with one with a slight hallux valgus deformity (below). Note that the outer side of the great toe joint (arrow)—the first metatarsophalangeal joint— is enlarged, and that the big toes angle away from one another. If the bursa over the involved joint is inflamed, it hurts, and it's a bunion.   Photo by Dale Durfee on skin moist from perspiration, an application of tincture of benzoin beneath tapings is always a good preventative practice. In fact, a daily painting of the feet with tincture of benzoin makes them tougher and less blister-prone; this practice, followed by a routine use of talc between the toes, is well worth the trouble. If you happen to use routinely a lot of adhesive tape, wait until your feet have cooled and dried before removing it, and save a little skin.

BUNIONS

Hallux valgus*—otherwise known as a "bunion"—is the most common painful deformity of the big toe. More correctly, the bunion is really an inflamed, thick-walled bursa that overlies the deformity. In dancers prone to this condition (a congenitally short first metatarsal can be a predisposing factor), pointe work forces deviation of the great toe toward the second with pressure induced enlargement of the outer side of the great toe joint. A similar process involving the little toe can lead to a painful enlargement on the outside of the foot, referred to as a "Tailor's bunion." Continued pressure and irritation to the area leads to an acutely inflamed bursa and consequent misery for the dancer; with further deviation of the toe, significant joint distortion as well as permanent degenerative changes can ensue.

Fortunately, even acutely inflamed bunions can settle down and go for long periods without causing any trouble. The best

---

* Visualize a dancer with a good-sized bunion on each foot, standing with feet together: the feet meet at the great toe joint while the toes head away from one another. If taken as analogous to genu valgus, the deformity seen in children when their knees come together, we might describe the condition as "knock-toed," a term I just made up and which will never be seen or heard outside of this footnote.

treatment, not surprisingly, is avoidance of pressure to the joint area. For the bunion plagued dancer, this can be a hard order to fill, since sometimes even getting shoes on at all is a lot to ask. Cutting wedges out of both sides and/or the back of the

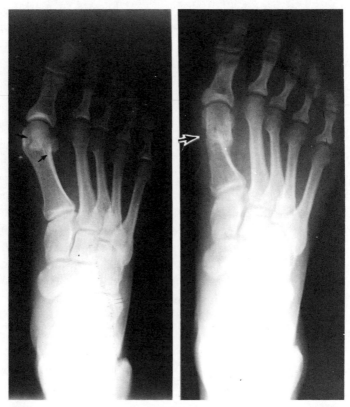

X-rays of a dancer's foot before (left) and after (right) surgical correction of the hallux valgus deformity. In this particular procedure, the deviation of the first metatarsal was corrected by a breaking and resetting of the bone (large arrow). The densities indicated by the small arrows are normal "extra" accessory bones of the foot.

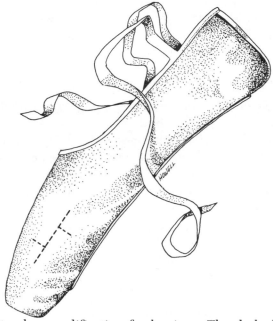

Pointe shoe modification for bunions. The dashed lines indicate the shoe incision to be made. The bulge that results when the foot is placed inside should be covered with a piece of moleskin.

shoe and sewing elastic in may be of some help. Another way to give the bunion room is to make an incision in the section of the toe box overlying the bunion, then cover the subsequent foot "bulge" with a piece of moleskin on the outside. If this is too noticeable for a performance, cut out an oval from the inside of the toe box with a linoleum knife, preserving the outer layer of satin (be careful to avoid rough edges, since this can cause irritation). The difficulty with this procedure is that the protruding foot is not well protected and is hence very vulnerable if accidently kicked or trod upon. For everyday use, common sense (or pain) should lead to the selection of wide, low-heeled street shoes.

Many dancers with hallux valgus routinely insert a piece of lamb's wool between the ends of the first two toes (placing it down at the base will only aggravate the problem); others strap a wide piece of adhesive tape across the top of the foot in order to pull the joint inwards. Both of these measures artificially correct the placement of the metatarsal bone and may help slightly if they can relieve some pressure. Remember that ice will usually provide some relief for the inflamed bunion—the best method is to apply moist heat to the area before dancing, then ice immediately after. An experienced New York podiatrist reports that the application of ten percent Ichthyol (an irritant) to the area, covered with gauze and left on overnight, can often bring about good results. For major bunion problems, some professional dancers employ custom-made latex rubber jackets which fit over the toe and have raised areas appropriately placed to relieve direct pressure on the bunion.

Incapacitating pain or the inability to wear shoes are the customary indications for surgical correction of the hallux valgus deformity. The surgical procedure selected must be individualized and depends on the patient's age, the degree of deformity, and the severity and duration of the symptoms. As a general rule, bunion surgery should be avoided by the dancer if at all possible. The so-called bumpectomy is a minor procedure in which the bone enlargement is tapered with an electric bone file under local anaesthesia; as it does not involve the opening of the joint, it averts possible toe deformity and the long rehabilitation made necessary by more invasive techniques. Of course, this treatment is by no means a satisfactory substitute for a more definitive procedure over the long haul, but it may be an adequate, dance-saving compromise for the ballerina.

CALLUSES

A callus is a thickening of the skin which comes about as a protective mechanism in response to friction and pressure. Although a certain amount of callus is healthy and normal for the ballerina, excess accumulation can often be the result of poor posture and weight bearing combined with faulty footwear. As callus tissue is inelastic, it tends to move as a mass and is thus vulnerable to tears and fissures. This cracking and torn skin can be painful and disabling to the dancer.

Excessive callus can be prevented by proper foot hygiene, appropriate apparel, and good dance technique. A routine of thorough foot cleansing, followed by filing off of excess callus with an emery file and application of a small amount of lanolin will pay dividends. Any time a dancer becomes aware of abnormal friction on the foot, she should immediately initiate preventive friction proofing, such as application of petroleum jelly or moleskin padding.

For those who are domestically oriented, a callus softener can be made by heating ½ cup castor oil, ½ cup paraffin wax, and one tablespoon of white soap chips or powder in a double boiler (do not place over direct heat) until blended. After cooling to about 100 degrees, stir in one teaspoon of sodium thiosulfate. Apply to the callus at bedtime and cover with gauze to protect the bed clothing. In the morning, the softener can be washed off with hot water. The mixture should be stored in a labeled container marked "Keep out of reach of children."

CORNS

And when too short the modish shoes are worn,
You'll judge the seasons by your shooting corns.
—JOHN GAY, *Trivia* (1716)

Corns are the most common dance-related foot problem, characteristically seen in female dancers and between the fourth and fifth toes. The fifth toe is often somewhat shorter than it should be in relation to the fourth, so that within the confines of the pointe shoe, the head of the small toe is pressed up against the base of its neighbor, stimulating overgrowth of skin in the irritated area.

Corns are localized callosities of two basic types. The hard

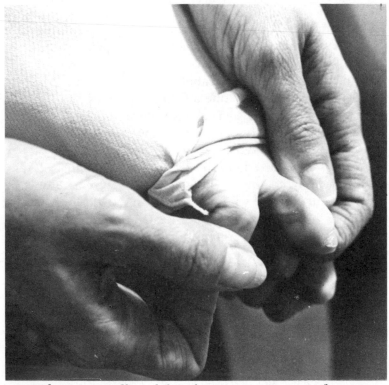

A dancer proudly exhibits her prize-winning soft corn (clavus molle), which, not surprisingly, is located between the fourth and fifth toes.

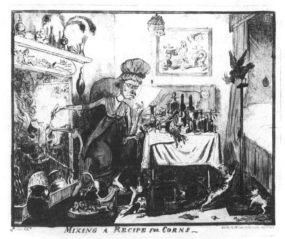

Mixing a Recipe for Corns

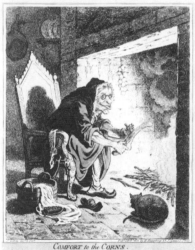

Comfort to the Corns.

Two interesting but ill-advised methods of dealing with
corns as depicted in prints by George Cruikshank (above,
published in London in 1835) and James Gillray (below,
published in London in 1800). —COURTESY OF THE LOGAN
CLENDENING HISTORY OF MEDICINE LIBRARY, THE
UNIVERSITY OF KANSAS MEDICAL CENTER

corn (*clavus durum*) is dense and rigid, is sharply demarcated from the normal tissue, and usually occurs on parts of the foot where the shoe exerts the greatest pressure—on the outside of the fifth toe and on top of the three middle toes. The soft corn (*clavus molle*) never gets the opportunity to become hard or cornified due to the constant moistness of its formative environment—between the toes. As corns press downward onto deeper, more sensitive skin, producing inflammation and pressure on nerve endings, they can be very tender and painful, particularly the hard variety, the more serious of the two types.

The best way to prevent disability is to prevent the corn by wearing a wide enough shoe with no pressure points, a realistic suggestion for a shopkeeper, maybe, but absurd for the dancer on pointe. Cutting wedges in the slipper—either at the middle on both sides or at the heel—and sewing in a small piece of elastic may ease pressure somewhat. Most dancers will have to resort to a wisp of lamb's wool wrapped around the toe, or better yet, a piece of 3/32-inch or thicker adhesive felt cut in the shape of a half-moon and placed around the upper edge of the corn (placing it directly on the corn will only increase the pressure). Occasionally, a corn—even the soft variety—will require minor surgical excision, particularly if there is an underlying bone spur promoting the corn formation.

There is no dearth of commercial medications for the alleged management of corns, but a specialist should always be consulted for a painful hard corn and for the paring or trimming of corns. More interesting to contemplate than employ are the numerous traditional folk remedies for corns, containing such ingredients as pine tar, saltpeter, tobacco extract, hickory bark ashes, vinegar, onions, mustard, lemon, brown sugar, celandine, Indian turnips, and nightshade berries boiled in hog's lard.

INGROWN TOENAILS

Abnormal pressure from short or narrow shoes (or just dancing on pointe) and improper trimming of toenails can lead to the toenail edge growing into the soft tissues of the skin, bringing about severe irritation and often infection. Ingrown toenails are one of those problems that can be seriously disabling to the dancer, and they should be avoided as much as possible by proper footwear and nail care.*

"Toenails should be cut straight across." Everyone knows this, but many dancers complain that straight nail edges cut into other toes when on demi-pointe; some conscientiously keep their nails very short and completely rounded and boast of no difficulties. Regardless, the safest bet is still to cut the nails fairly close to the quick and straight across, or even a little concave. If one insists on keeping the nails slightly rounded, they should never be long enough to contact the skin on either side of the nail bed. Trim the nails often—this will also help eliminate the problem of breaking and the bother of cutting the nail down in gradual increments when it has been allowed to grow too long (some dancers claim that cutting off too much nail can be painful on pointe initially because of the inadequacy of the toe callus). And finally, if you're inclined to pick nervously at your nails, keep your shoes on as much as possible!

There are ways of dealing with ingrown toenails besides gritting one's teeth. Although sometimes partial removal of the nail by a podiatrist or physician is required, removal of the entire nail is seldom warranted or necessary for the dancer. Probably the best home remedy is hot soaks two or three times a day, followed by the insertion (not jamming) of a thin piece of lamb's wool or foam rubber under the edge of the affected nail

---

* This disability may be listed more romantically as *unguis incarnatus* on the application form for workmen's compensation.

(this lifts the nail slightly, protects the tender skin beneath, and guides the nail as it grows forward). This procedure should be continued until the ingrown nail has grown out and the symptoms are gone. Some people suggest filing a groove or cutting a small wedge down the center of the nail, theoretically allowing the nail to buckle slightly and relieve the pressure from the edges. Even if this provides some relief, it is probably useless in the long run, as the cut has no effect on nail growth (from the base) and might even cause artificial curling of the nail. The worst thing to do is simply to cut off the offending corner of nail; this allows the skin in front of the nail edge to press against the nail as it grows and only aggravates the condition.

For quick, temporary relief of pain, those troopers who have to go on stage and teeth-grit under the smile can use Xylocaine jelly or ointment, but they should remember to leave easy access to the toe through the tights, since one application won't last long enough to get a dancer through an entire performance.*

BREAKING TOENAILS

Broken or cracked nails are usually caused by jamming the nail, often by a dancer rolling forward on pointe. The easy way to eliminate the problem is simply to keep the toenails trimmed short enough at all times. In the case of breakage, there is generally no cause for removing the entire nail. Partial nail plate removal, if required, can be performed by a podiatrist, who will file the remaining nail edge smooth, paint with gentian violet or some other antiseptic, and cover with adhe-

---

* Don't be misled into thinking that this topical anaesthetic has more than limited usefulness—overuse tends to cause maceration of the skin.

sive tape. Continuing to dance will not hamper correct nail regrowth any more than the damage caused by the nail's breaking in the first place. Nails should always be kept clean along the free edge and sides, since an infection of the nail bed can develop if the neighboring skin is broken.

For those who like fingernail hardeners, try this recipe the next time you're in the kitchen making slice-and-bake cookies: Mix three tablespoons of water with one tablespoon of glycerin and one teaspoon of powdered alum. Coat the nails with the solution at night by dipping or by applying with a small brush. Remove the residue in the morning with alcohol and cotton. The solution should be kept in an appropriately labeled container marked "Keep out of reach of children."

PART THREE

General Specifics
(From the Bottom Up)

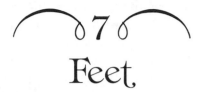

Feet

Your pedal extremities really are obnoxious.
—Fats Waller

Feet are at the bottom of it all, physically, spiritually, and every other possible way.* Undeservedly, they are the object of abuse and disregard—the dancer's foot has to be strong, supple, and practically as sensitive as the hand, not to mention beautiful (beautiful, that is, at some distance and covered up, since many dancers' feet look like something the cat dragged in). Until recently, I was under the mistaken impression that feet were aesthetic boors; that they were unable to grasp subtleties or appreciate any sensations other than those produced by a stubbed toe or hot asphalt (both instances of pain, a very primitive response). My few attempts at picking up things with my feet or playing the piano with them as a child were always thwarted; consequently, I, like many others, considered them stupid and unrefined. Then came the turnabout. Out of curiosity, I asked a dancer with the New York City Ballet the all-important question: "What do you stuff in your toe shoes?" (It has become an unconscious habit with me to ask this question as routinely as others might inquire about a favorite color, star sign, or least favorite vegetable). Her reply was quite

---

* Take my word for it, this is well documented in myth, literature, and anthropology. For example, "Kiss my feet" is as much a reflection on the low esteem of the feet as the person addressed.

precise: "Three squares of toilet paper, single ply." This state-
ment of fact was delivered with such conviction that one re-
ceived the impression that to sneak in an extra half of a square
would be an act of sabotage. My mouth dropped in amazement.
Here at last was a discriminative foot, a pedal epicure, a verita-
ble prodigy.

"Any particular brand?" I asked.

"Just whatever they have around here," she answered,
undercutting my enthusiasm a bit. "I'll use Kleenex in a pinch,
but with too much stuffing, I can't feel and manipulate my
toes—there isn't enough intimate contact with the floor."

Admittedly, I still can't rid myself of an ever-so-slight linger-
ing contempt for feet; but I willingly concede that these beasts
of burden—harassed and harangued by the dancer—deserve a
lot of credit, ugly or not.

ANATOMY

The foot consists of the tarsal bones (the talus, calcaneus,
navicular, cuboid, and three cuneiforms), five metatarsals, and
fourteen phalanges—three in each toe except in the little piggy
that went to market, which only has two bones.* For those who
are mathematically oriented, that comes to a total of 26 bones
per foot, 52 per dancer, and in the neighborhood of 4,680 for a
good-sized company. The bones are arranged in such a way as
to form two principal arches; the preservation of this architec-
tural structure is the responsibility of the binding long and
short ligaments and the muscles and tendons that pass under-
foot. The longitudinal arches are present on the inside as well
as the outside of the foot (the inner, or medial, arch is much
higher and more elastic than its outer solid and only slightly

---

* Physician's note: the piggy that went to market is the great toe.

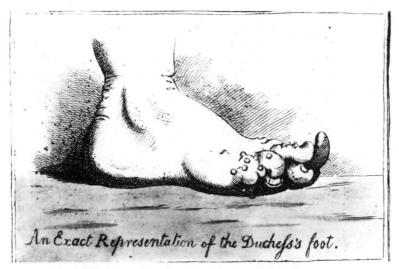

An Exact Representation of the Duchess's foot.

A vivid representation of the Duchess's foot, published in 1792 in London. Although the identities of the artist and the particular Duchess remain a mystery to this day, rumor has it that she danced. —COURTESY OF THE LOGAN CLENDENING HISTORY OF MEDICINE LIBRARY, THE UNIVERSITY OF KANSAS MEDICAL CENTER

elevated counterpart); the transverse arch runs across the forefoot and forms the dome in the middle of the foot that should appear when one is standing with both feet together.

ARCHES

There are two extremes of longitudinal arch elevation, *pes planus,* or flatfoot, and *pes cavus,* high longitudinal arch. The acquired flatfoot is usually flexible, assuming a flattened position when weight bearing, but forming an arch with movement of the muscles or when on pointe. This may be associated with generalized ligamentous laxity and excessive mobility in joints such as the hips, knees, and elbow, although a dancer can be hyperextended elsewhere and paradoxically have tight feet, the so-called spoons. Characteristically, a flat-footed person will "toe out" when walking normally.

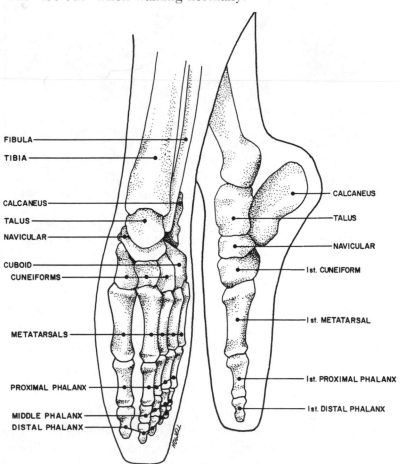

The foot skeleton.

With an unusually high longitudinal arch (also called "claw-foot" or "hollow foot"), abnormal stresses are placed on the instep, ball of the foot, and heel. The foot is shortened by the high arch convexity and the toes are clawed; heavy callus forms on top of the toes and under the metatarsal heads particularly, as well as on the ball of the foot and the heel. Although this type of foot may be without symptoms, pain when it exists is usually a result of excess pressure on the metatarsals or of fatigue. Wherever the foot structure fits in the scheme of things, the dancer's arches must always stand on their own, since ballet slippers and pointe shoes will provide virtually nothing in the way of support.

Unfortunately, a foot cannot be all things to all dancers. A very high-arched foot may be especially beautiful to look at, but it will not be nearly as sturdy as a more tightly knit foot; it may fatigue much more easily and may even have the tendency to roll over on pointe. Among high-arched feet, an arch which begins in the middle of the foot is probably stronger than, while still as aesthetically pleasing as, an arch that begins practically at the ankle joint. Regardless of these generalizations, every dancer is quite certain if her feet are "good" or "bad"; it doesn't take any knowledge of anatomy to know whether they hurt or not (just try to convince a dancer with a sturdy arch and the ideal "square" foot how perfect her feet are for dance while she is soaking them).

MOVEMENTS

All movements of the foot are performed by a series of muscles which, with one exception, attach below the knee at one end and to various bones of the foot at the other, and four layers of muscles contained in the foot itself. To make things complicated, most of these muscles have more than one action.

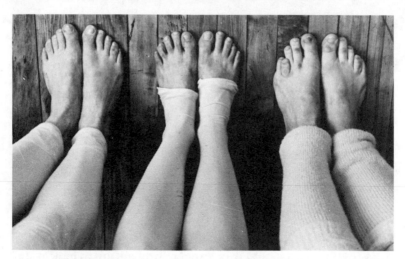

In comparing these bizarre appendages used frequently by dancers—called feet—it is interesting to note variations in relative toe lengths. Incidentally, in an ugly foot competition, the pair on the far right came in second only to the Duchess's (see p. 75). Photo by Dale Durfee

The movements can, however, be sorted out individually.

Plantar flexion is pointing the foot downward; the opposite move, elevating the front part of the foot, is *dorsiflexion* (*dorsum* referring to the top of the foot, *plantar* to the surface that comes in contact with the ground). Raising the inner border of the foot is, in medical jargon, *inversion;* the lift of the outer border is called *eversion.* Turning the forefoot in toward its neighbor is called *adduction;* turning it away is *abduction.* And for the finale: a combination of adduction and inversion (with a bit of plantar flexion) is called *supination;* abduction with eversion (and dorsiflexion) is called *pronation.* To help remember this one, think of a flat-footed person walking duck-footed—an example of the pronated foot.

Obviously, pointing the foot is the equivalent action to lifting the heel off the ground with the foot on the floor; hence, being on pointe is plantar flexion (similarly, the foot is in dorsiflexion at the bottom of a demi-plié). In rising on the toes, 95 percent of the lift is provided by the two calf muscles that end in the Achilles tendon: the superficial gastrocnemius and the underlying soleus. The gastrocnemius (the only muscle working the foot that originates above the knee) is also involved with knee flexion; however, with the knee bent, it loses its effectiveness on the foot and the soleus becomes the more important plantar flexor.* Parenthetically, an accessory muscle for plantar flexion is the flexor digitorum longus. Since it originates on the back side of the tibia and inserts on the base of the distal phalanges of the four outer toes, it also causes the toes to flex in a gripping manner. This anatomical gem is only pertinent if you have ever wondered why the toes have a tendency to curl when pointing the foot.

The principal dorsiflexor is the tibialis anterior; it gets the heels to the ground when rising from a grand plié. In addition to dorsiflexion, this muscle causes inversion of the foot, as does its counterpart, the tibialis posterior. Both of these muscles are responsible for pulling the leg over the foot while balancing on one leg; their tendons pass around the inner ankle and under the foot and are important supporters of the arch. Inverters as well as everters act as foot stabilizers with the foot on the ground; muscles which primarily evert the ankle are the peroneus longis and peroneus brevis. Running along the outer

---

* This is easy to appreciate. Stand on demi-pointe with straight knees and feel the muscular contour of either calf. Now lift that same leg into passé (keep the foot pointed), and you can feel the change—the major responsibility for keeping the foot pointed has shifted from the gastrocnemius to its partner, the soleus. Incidentally, both muscles together are known as the *triceps surae.*

side of the calf, they are ineffective plantar flexors themselves, but they evert the foot most successfully when the foot is pointing.

The four layers of short muscles on the underside of the foot work as a group; their chief concern being to change the foot's shape. They also serve as an added source of strength for the longitudinal arch, help to propel the foot in walking, and hold the toes firmly to the ground when standing. Unlike other muscles which pass over a joint and effect a lever-type action, these unpretentious muscles function merely by contracting for contraction's sake, changing shape without influencing joint motion. To truly use and develop these muscles, then, force must be applied against some fixed object to allow them to come into full play. The most convenient source of resistance for the bottom of the foot is none other than the floor, which is why "using the floor" is so important. Pushing down on battement tendu and striking the ground with frappé are not for naught.

TECHNICAL PROBLEMS

With these simplified basics in mind, we can consider what is going on mechanically with the most common foot problems of dancers. With proper weight bearing, the distribution of force forms more or less a triangle on the bottom of the foot (think of a healthy footprint). Correct transmission of the weight becomes much more difficult with the feet turned out 180 degrees. If a turn-out comes from the knee or the ankle rather than the hips, the proper alignment of foot to leg to thigh is lost, and a disproportionate amount of weight comes over the inner side of the foot, causing it to roll inwards (eversion). This bulging over the inner border of the foot can lead to irreversible stretching of the ligaments (with accompanying acute or

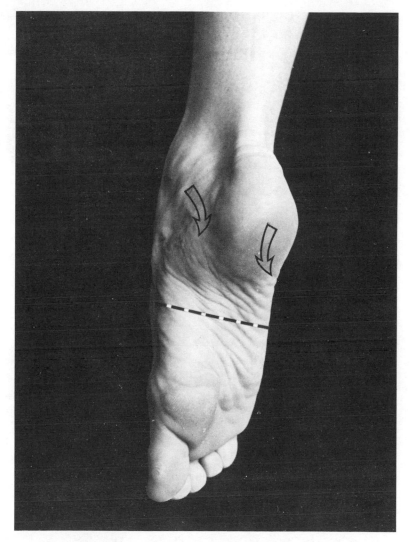

The arches of the foot: medial longitudinal (inside arrow);
lateral longitudinal (outside arrow); transverse (dashed line).
Photo by William H. Batson

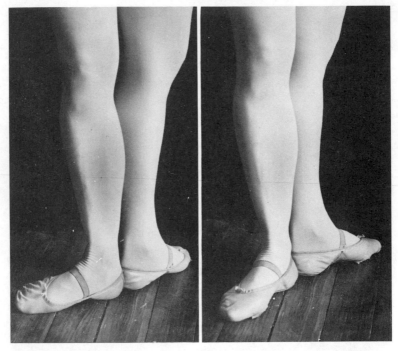

A comparison of "rolling-in" of the foot (left) and proper positioning (right).   Photos by William H. Batson

chronic flat feet), as well as tendon strain. Many feel that rolling (and, as you will see, sickling), be it the result of forcing turn-out or any other cause, is largely responsible for chronic tendon problems (particularly of the Achilles and posterior tibialis tendons), since a malposition produces malalignment or "bowing" of the involved tendon. With rolling, the battle for foot stabilization is obviously being won by the everters over the inverters (if you're a roller, check for a well-developed peroneal group bulge on the outer side of the leg), but it takes

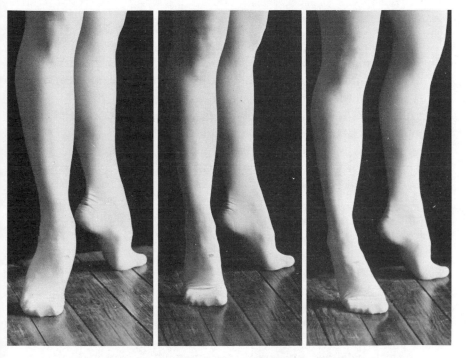

Two types of sickling on demi-pointe: on the far left, the
eversion variety (what most probably call "sickling-in");
on the far right, the inversion variety. The feet in the middle
are correctly situated.   Photos by William H. Batson

more than overworking the inverters to compensate for the
problem. A conscious attempt to combat rolling by forcing
inversion of the feet usually causes the great toe to lift off the
ground, shifting the weight to the outside of the foot. This can
lead to bruising of the outside metatarsals as well as to arch
strain, not to mention its disastrous effect on proper placement. The best way to combat a roll is to work on turn-out from

the hip (and settle for less rather than push it) and to develop the intrinsic foot muscles with appropriate foot exercises.

A similar problem to rolling is sickling, which occurs on demi-pointe. The foot and ankle can either roll inward, placing a strain on the longitudinal arch and the great toe, or they can roll to the outside, in which case the strain is placed on the outer ligaments of the foot and ankle (the tendons passing on either side of the ankle will likewise be strained). Confusingly, some people refer to the first situation as "sickling in" (which seems most acceptable to me), while others call it "sickling out," and vice versa for the latter. The choice of terms is ambiguous—when the ankle and mid-foot bulge away or "out," the foot is "inverted" and the heels point "in"; thus it depends on the frame of reference. Many dance instructors use the term more loosely, referring to a working foot as "sickled" whenever the heel is poorly positioned; for example, if the heel is not pushed adequately forward in a tendu en avant or a passé, or the foot is not "winged" in attitude or arabesque derrière. The preferred usage of the word comes about with proper muscle control, balance, and good technique, which eliminate it altogether from the dancer's vocabulary.

MARCH FRACTURE

The term "march fracture" refers to a fracture of the metatarsal bone that is the consequence of accumulated impact and shock, an insult most characteristically suffered by foot-stomping military personnel during long treks. Dancers may have more finesse than soldiers, but they aren't any less susceptible to these hairline fractures of the shafts of the second or third metatarsals. Pain and tenderness are particularly associated with jumping; the symptoms subside with rest but resume with activity, which may additionally produce swelling

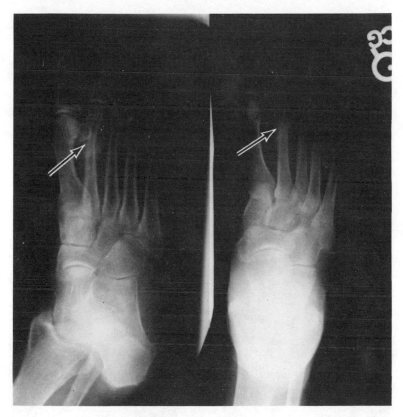

You may appreciate that something is amiss in the second metatarsal (not just because of the arrow!) because of a circular fluffy area of increased density around the bony shaft. What you see is another type of "callus," an unorganized meshwork of bone that is a normal reaction and actually part of the healing process of a bone fracture. The underlying fracture in this case is a march fracture, and with straining, you may be able to make out part of the remaining fracture line. The sharply defined bony density at the end of the first metatarsal is a normal accessory bone.

and redness. Initial X-rays may reveal nothing, and by the time bony reaction confirms the diagnosis on film, the dancer may be already almost completely healed and resuming a tolerable amount of dancing. As the fracture heals spontaneously without the need for splinting or taping, treatment generally entails no jumping for three weeks to a month, as the symptoms dictate; but there is always the possibility that more restrictive measures may be necessary.

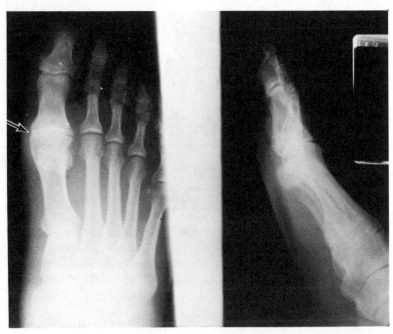

The increased density of white in the area of the first metatarsophalangeal joint is indicative of arthritic changes, or hallux rigidus. Note that the involved joint space is relatively narrower than its counterparts (arrow).

HALLUX RIGIDUS

This form of arthritis involves the joint between the foot and the great toe (the first metatarsophalangeal joint), a joint subjected to tremendous stresses in dancing. It usually begins in adolescence and is more common in males, presumedly because the male dancer wears soft, tightly fitting shoes all of the time and has more mild continual trauma to the big toe as a result of jumping. Continued irritation to the big toe joint leads to joint enlargement and inflammation; gradually, over a period of time, the toe can become permanently rigid. Pain and restriction of motion at this joint is a severe disability in that it limits the height of demi-pointe and seriously impairs jumping. More generally, every step normally requires unhindered extension (dorsiflexion) at the great toe.

Specialists may suggest helpful forms of treatment for both the early and the chronic condition. Acute flare-ups are common and should be treated with great respect and care, including not only complete rest, but also manipulation by a trained physical therapist. When the condition is severe and osteoarthritic changes have occurred, surgery is usually necessary; reportedly—as far as certain male dancers are concerned—surgical procedures have been successful.

HAMMER TOE

Cramped toes can eventually lead to toe deformity, hammer toe being a good example in the dancer. In this condition, the first toe bone points upwards, while the second and third phalanges are flexed downward. This deformity is especially prevalent in the second toe, which is often slightly longer than the great toe and hence is bent down at the end when on pointe. Additionally, hallux valgus can cause the great toe to encroach upon and under its neighbor, again causing it to hammer. The ends of hammered toes are typically well callused, as are the top surfaces from pressure against the shoe (this is often contributory to the development of hard corns on the tops of the three middle toes).

Once hammering develops, there are no corrective exercises, and manual stretching of the flexed toes is not effective. A one-half-inch-wide strip of adhesive tape, alternately running under and over adjacent toes at their base, may be a somewhat helpful strapping technique.

TOE SPRAIN

Jamming the toes against a more worthy opponent (such as the floor) is an occupational hazard of the dancer and is generally the cause of toe sprains. Although symptoms usually disappear after standard treatment, if the great toe is involved, attempts to resume working are often accompanied by the recurrence of pain, swelling, and disability. The dancer must thus be prepared to limit the toe's weight-bearing activities for as long as ten days to two weeks, although strapping may provide enough stability to permit less restriction. For each of the other toes, taping to one or more of its healthy neighbors usually provides enough immobilization to allow unimpeded dancing while neither prolonging nor accelerating the normal healing process (which will proceed along at its own pace for about ten to twelve days). It goes without saying that the injury should always be appraised for the possibility of fracture.

BRUISED GREAT TOE

Not uncommonly, a dancer on pointe will jam her great toe in a way which causes bleeding under the nail and produces pressure build-up and pain (especially if she has the tendency to roll over and is not properly manicured). A podiatrist can quickly and easily remedy this problem by drilling a small hole into the nail, a painless procedure which allows the trapped blood to escape, thereby relieving the pressure. After a hot soak in water and antiseptic, the dancer can immediately go back on pointe without any difficulty—an otherwise impossible task with a painfully bruised great toe.

PLANTAR FASCIAL STRAIN

Landing from leaps and jumps can triple or even quadruple the forces that the foot normally encounters. These jarring stresses can strain the plantar fascia, a sheet of fibrous tissue that extends from the heel to the bases of the toes, investing the muscles and other structures under the sole of the foot and assisting in maintaining the arch. Damage to this tough membrane causes pain and limitation of movement, and is considered by many physicians to be one of the most common serious problems of dancers—stubborn, obstinate, and often difficult to manage. Some physicians employ strapping techniques; some use ultrasound; and others modify ballet footwear with small inserts or heel lifts. Generally, strapping is impractical for the dancer, and many will not tolerate pads in their slippers. The specialist's recommendations will almost certainly include a reduction in training schedule, application of heat or cold, and appropriate non-weight-bearing exercises. If slipper inserts aren't feasible, taking classes in a jazz shoe may be more practical, and a supporting device can be used in street shoes, if nowhere else.

FOOT SOAKS

Find a dancer's feet out of pointe shoes, and they're probably soaking in a basin. What to put in the basin? Dancers' testimonials abound for the "soothing and inflammation-reducing" powers of Burows solution (aluminum acetate solution occasionally stabilized with a pinch of boric acid). The principal medical use for Burows is in the treatment of certain dermatologic conditions, in which it acts by a combination of detergent, antiseptic, astringent, and heat-dispersing effects. It's an institution among dancers, but if overused it can be very irritating to the skin and cause cracks between the toes (as can alum, another astringent used in soaks to harden the skin of the feet). When soaking in Burows, dilute it with twenty to thirty parts of water, or soak a towel in the diluted mixture, wrap it around the foot, and cover with Saran Wrap.

Though my intent is not to destroy a sacred cow, soaking in hot water with some Ivory or Lux flakes may be just as miracle-performing and a lot less irritating. The skin-hardening effects of Burows can be obtained by painting the foot daily with tincture of benzoin, allowing five minutes to dry, and giving the foot a good once-over with talc. The residue can easily be removed with alcohol. Application of the tincture is also helpful before using adhesive tape or bandages—it protects the skin, cuts down tape rash, and makes removal of the tape easier.

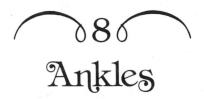

Ankles

The ankle is often the focus of problems, either indirectly, because of the tendons that pass in front, behind, and on either side, or directly, because of its susceptibility to sprain. As if continual jumping, with its unavoidable twists and slips, weren't enough reason for sprain, it so happens that the ankle is least stable when the foot is pointed. For the dancer then, the ankle is in its most vulnerable position most of the time.

The joint itself is between the tibia, fibula, and talus. Although the fibula is not a weight-bearing bone and is not directly involved in the knee joint, it forms a vital part of the ankle.* The knob on the outer side of the ankle is in fact a projection of the fibula (called the lateral malleolus), while the bony projection on the inside (the medial malleolus) is part of the tibia. The talus, the first foot bone to receive the weight from the upper body, fits snugly in between. When the foot is in a demi-plié (dorsiflexed), the talus is sandwiched in such a way that there is no movement from side to side. This isn't the case with the pointed foot; there's enough give to either side to cause trouble. Characteristically, ankle sprains occur when the foot rolls over towards the outside and is twisted, overstretch-

---

* Next time you're chomping away on the drumstick of a chicken, take note of that long, skinny sharp bone, and the origin of the word will make sense. In the Latin, *fibula* refers to the needle of a brooch or the tongue of a buckle. The relationship of the fibula to the tibia is that of the needle of the brooch to the brooch, the fibula being the needle.

ing the outside lateral collateral ligament of the ankle (the "inversion" sprain). The other principal supporting ligament of the ankle is on the inside and is called the deltoid. Although this ligament will be stretched with eversion forces (the foot turning under to the inside), it is so strong that part of the ankle bone will usually be broken away (avulsion) before the ligament tears.

Odds are that if you ever sprain anything, it will be the ankle. Remember that the internal bleeding from injury distends the joints and overstretches the ligaments, and also favors the development of adhesions. And no matter how great your personal physician's diagnostic prowess, a swollen ankle only complicates an already tough assessment problem. Appropriate and immediate use of cold, compression, and elevation may give you less time on the sidelines to idly knit warm-ups.

ACHILLES TENDINITIS

The Achilles tendon is figuratively as well as literally the dancer's Achilles heel.* First described by Galen in the second century A.D., this calf muscle tendon is used ubiquitously by the dancer and is extremely susceptible to overstretching and strain.† Not only is an improperly cared for strain susceptible to becoming a chronic bother, but prolonged, nontraumatic,

---

* We all know that Achilles was smitten by Paris during the siege of Troy by a well-placed cheap-shot to the heel, the only part of his anatomy left vulnerable after his dip as a child in the legendary river Styx. The Trojan could obviously have done away with his enemy much more deviously by encouraging the Grecian to take up ballet.

† Galen (A.D. 130–200), one of the giants in medical history, was also team doc for the gladiators.

irritative stresses can also result in Achilles tendinitis. In fact, more often than not, the condition appears with overwork suddenly and with no explanation, particularly in those with very tight or very narrow tendons. Since the problem can often be fairly resistant to treatment, and since avoidance of stretching the tendon is virtually incompatible with dancing, it's no wonder that tendinitis is so prevalent and bothersome in the dance world.

The inflammatory process involves the tendon or the loose connective tissue about the tendon (hence the term Achilles paratendinitis); since the *tendo Achilles* is not surrounded by a true tendon sheath, the term Achilles tendosynovitis (inflammation of the synovium between the tendon and its sheath) is inaccurate and misleading. Aside from the unavoidable dancing stresses that may lead to this condition, culpability appears to be empirically cast upon hard floors, sickling and rolling of the foot, and that old reliable, forcing turn-out.

Pain will result from any forcible pushing of the foot against the floor (which may mean with every step taken), but the area may also be tender to touch. The preferred treatment is complete rest (with the condition, hopefully, clearing up in from one to three weeks), but so much for dreaming. Most dancers will stubbornly refuse the rest; some will dance for years with chronic recurring tendon problems. Of course, many dancers will compromise with a brief inactive period, but returning to work, even with minimal discomfort, usually will bring back all the symptoms immediately (especially if a technical problem is contributing to the disorder to begin with).

For those dancers who take stock in the German proverb "If I rest, I rust," certain measures may help to win what, practically speaking, may become a losing battle. If possible, ease the stretch on the tendon by using heel lifts in both slippers or, better yet, by wearing jazz shoes. For purists who can't dance with such altered footwear, at least wear heeled shoes (or use heel pads) for street wear. Raising the dancing heel is probably a more feasible and less cumbersome alternative than athletic strapping, which some will recommend. Various physicians may suggest shortwave, ultrasound, muscle relaxants, and other therapeutic procedures, but no one technique appears to be any more definitive than stabs in the dark that may prove fruitful. Contrast baths seem fairly highly recommended, as does the standard use of moist heat before, followed by application of ice or cold water after, dancing. Hordes of dancers are walking advertisements for the most prevalent therapeutic aid: Saran Wrap. Rumor has it that rubbing cooking oil on the afflicted part and wrapping with a warm, moist washcloth (wrapped in Saran and kept warm with a heat pad) is beneficial, although I can't speculate if, or why, cooking oil should have more miraculous effects than the heat itself.

One last word of warning: local injections of steroids or anaesthetics are unwarranted; although providing symptomatic relief, they cause no immediate alteration of the actual inflammatory process, and this practice has been suspiciously associated with cases of spontaneous rupture of the tendon. Dramatic local relief can lead to the resumption of overly vigorous activity, and may mean conversion of a partial tear to a complete one.

ACHILLES BURSITIS

Friction from shoes against the heel can lead to irritation and subsequent inflammation of the bursa located between the Achilles tendon and the skin, resulting in pain and tenderness that may be confused with Achilles tendinitis. The two conditions may usually be distinguished by the fact that the pain of achillobursitis will more likely be brought on by local pressure than by active contraction of the calf muscles, but this is not always clear-cut. Aside from ill-fitting shoes, sliding the heel along the bar à la seconde probably doesn't help any. Since continued irritation can lead to a chronically thickened bursa and thickened skin, as well as to the deposition of calcium (not to mention the tendency for blisters to form in this area), pressure and friction to the area should be alleviated to as great an extent as possible. Moleskin over the heel area can cut back on friction, but it doesn't do much for the pressure. Here again, the old trick of cutting wedges in the slippers and sewing in elastic may prove helpful. Oftentimes, aching in the Achilles area is due to nothing more than pressure from the pointe shoe ribbon. Cut the ribbon at the section that normally winds around the heel and sew in a one-to-two-inch piece of elastic. Relieving the pressure in this way may make the problem disappear.

ACHILLES TENDON RUPTURE

This is probably the most dreaded and feared injury that can befall a ballet dancer. Ambroise Paré, the father of French surgery, described in 1575 an "affect of the large tendon of the heel," which "oft times is rent or torn by a small occasion without any sign of injury or solution of continuity apparent on the outside as by a little jump, the slipping aside of the foot, the too nimble getting on horseback, or the slipping of the foot out of the stirrup in mounting into the saddle. When this chance happens, it will give a crack like a coachman's whip; above the head where the tendon is broken the depressed cavity may be felt with your finger; there is great pain in the part and party is not able to go."

The fact that an apparently minor provocation can wreak such havoc accounts for the paranoia; however, the instigating insult is in every sense that single added straw that will send the camel to the orthopedist—that slight extra stretch to a maximally stretched tendon, a forced stretch to a relaxed or unprepared tendon, or a direct blow to a tendon that, once again, will simply stretch no more. With a complete tear, early surgical repair is a necessity. Immobilization in plaster will last approximately a month, to be followed by gradual rehabilitation. Prophets of doom consider this injury equivalent to retirement for the dancer, and although this may not be the case, a return to major dancing with heavy jumping remains questionable.

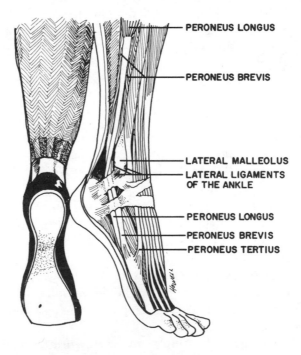

The ankle and vicinity (lateral view).

Common sense and precautions can help avert this dance-disaster. Routine stretching and warm-up of the calves and Achilles should always be high priority; an Achilles strain should be treated with the respect it deserves; and superficial temporary relief for Achilles tendon problems by injections should absolutely never be considered.

DANCER'S HEEL

Dancers who do a lot of pointe work on a hard floor will sometimes develop pain above the heel bone (calcaneus) in the

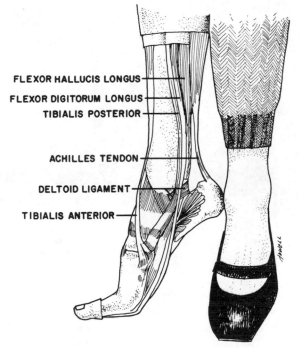

FLEXOR HALLUCIS LONGUS
FLEXOR DIGITORUM LONGUS
TIBIALIS POSTERIOR

ACHILLES TENDON

DELTOID LIGAMENT

TIBIALIS ANTERIOR

The ankle and vicinity (medial view).

area of the Achilles tendon; this condition, commonly referred to as "dancer's heel," is apparently caused by inflammation secondary to trauma in the joint between the calcaneus and the talus. The pain is brought about by pointing the foot, making pointe work with knees properly straightened quite difficult. Since standard physical therapy techniques sometimes have little effect, the most appropriate treatment is rest, which,

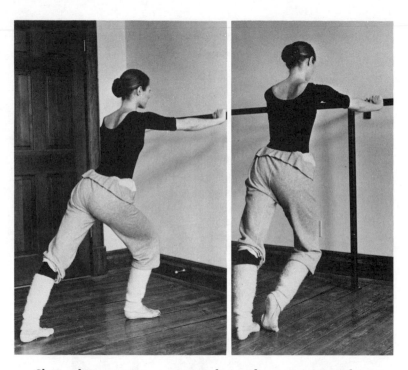

Shown here are some commonly used warm-up stretches of the Achilles' tendon. A few good demi-pliés will serve the purpose; or, if a staircase is handy, stand on the edge of a step with the ball of the foot, then slowly rise up and lower. Photos by William H. Batson

practically speaking, means working flat-footed or rising only so far as not to cause pain.

OS TRIGONUM

The os trigonum is a small bone which may be either separate from or fused to (in which case it makes a small "lip") the

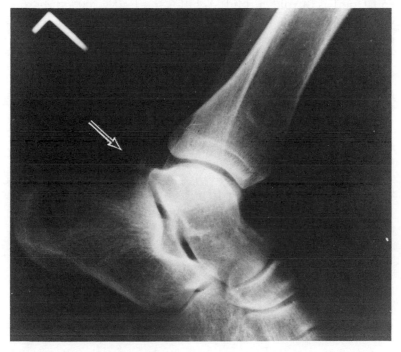

The small piece of bone that forms a sort of "lip" at the end of the talus is an os trigonum, a normal anatomical variation that can occasionally be a pain for the dancer on pointe (arrow).

rear part of the ankle bone (talus). Usually absent, it is a normal anatomical variation, a completely functionless structure which in the dancer may impede function. On full pointe, the back upper surface of the calcaneus normally comes up almost to touch the lower end of the tibia. If the os trigonum is present, it may form a block between the two bones, nipping soft tissue structures, causing inflammation, and restricting full plantar flexion. The pain behind the ankle may again be misconstrued as the old faithful, Achilles tendinitis, a good reason why persistent pain behind the ankle joint should be evaluated by X-ray to appropriately elucidate the cause. Surgical removal of the bone relieves the symptoms and entails approximately a three-month recovery period. It is important to note that the preferred surgical approach is from the inside (medial) rather than the outside (lateral), since the latter method can result in adhesions of the peroneal tendons and may require many months of rehabilitation before the full range of movement is restored.

Dancers with the os trigonum may be perfectly symptom-free, particularly those who do not have adequate flexion to get them into trouble, or those with supple enough feet to compensate for the slight loss of flexion at the ankle joint and still attain a good pointe.

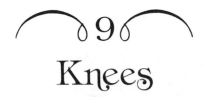

Knees

The knee is a complicated and very strong joint, one which rarely should give the dancer trouble—rarely, that is, if the dancer can avoid rolling over on pointe, ligament laxity, forcing turn-out, kneeling, degenerative changes, and plain old twists and mishaps.

Articulations of the knee joint involve the femur, the tibia, the kneecap, and knee cartilage. The two oval cartilage pieces, called menisci, assist in shock absorption and provide a slightly deeper socket for the joint. The principal ligaments include the collateral ligaments (on both inner and outer sides), which provide lateral stability, and the cruciate ligaments (inside the joint capsule), which provide front-to-back stabilization. The greatest source of stabilizing strength, however, comes from the bracing muscles of the thigh and calf. Since these are also the only supporting structures whose strength can be improved, they are the first line of defense against knee stresses. The powerful quadriceps group undergoes atrophy with disuse faster than any other muscle in the body; with prolonged layoffs, inadequate support from this key muscle may allow instability of the knee and increase the likelihood of injury.

With a completely straight knee, both the cruciate and the collateral ligaments are taut. Semiflexion results in the relaxation of the cruciates as well as of the lateral collateral, leaving only the medial collateral ligament as the primary supporter. Since a small amount of side movement is thus possible when the knee is bent, the traditional comparison of knee motion to

Structure of the knee.

LATERAL (FIBULAR)
COLLATERAL LIGAMENT

MEDIAL (TIBIAL)
COLLATERAL LIGAMENT

PATELLAR LIGAMENT

INFRAPATELLAR BURSA

DEEP INFRAPATELLAR BURSA

MEDIAL MENISCUS
(CARTILAGE)

LATERAL MENISCUS
(CARTILAGE)

PREPATELLAR BURSA

PATELLA

SUPRAPATELLAR BURSA

GASTROCNEMIUS

QUADRICEPS

FEMUR

the back-and-forth action of a hinge is a gross simplification (ronds de jambe en l'air demonstrate this capability for rotary movement). In fact, because of the contours of the articulating surfaces in the joint, there is always a certain degree of rotary motion, slightly outward with extension and inward with flexion.

Because the bent knee has the least stability, the vast majority of knee injuries will occur with the knee in some degree of flexion and weight bearing. A poor landing from a jump is a perfect setup for producing more rotational stresses than can be tolerated at the joint. Although a knee sprain can be the dramatic result of a single twist of the body with the leg bent and fixed to the floor, many knee injuries will be more insidious, the result of repeated twisting insults and stresses that cause a general laxity of the ligaments and make the knee more vulnerable.

"SCREWING" THE KNEE AND OTHER FAULTS

How can some of these twisting stresses be avoided? Primarily with good technique and adequate strength of the supporting musculature. Probably the biggest pitfall is failure to keep the knees directly over the feet in pliés. The most common mistake is "screwing" the knee, a flaw particularly prevalent in male dancers who lack adequate hip flexibility and consequently force turn-out from the knees down.

Characteristically, this is done in the following manner: Suppose a male dancer can only turn out properly about 130 degrees of external rotation; taking advantage of the side-to-side movement allowed with knee flexion, he makes up the difference by rotating the tibia on the femur while in a demi-plié, then straightens the knees with the feet fixed in the turned-out position. The medial collateral ligament takes the stress, which is compounded with knee bending because the malalignment alters proper weight distribution (an excess going to the inside of the knee, particularly when foot rolling is also a factor). Theoretically, "screwing" the knee may directly affect the kneecap because of the abnormal wear and tear that comes from the uneven pull on the patella. Not surprisingly, male dancers who began dancing in their middle to late teens (a late age) often show significant laxity of the knee ligaments as a result of this practice.

Even with a good turn-out, some dancers have a tendency to fall inwards when rising from a plié, which also puts stress on the medial collateral ligament. Sitting at the bottom of the plié is another subtle way to torture the knee, as is rolling over forward on pointe. A properly executed rond de jambe en l'air ends with a strong extension and straightening of the joint to a stable position—performing them à terre with a relaxed knee is obviously detrimental, in that it allows rotational stresses that would otherwise be avoided with a straight, secure knee. Dancers who overuse resin may also get into trouble—if the foot is stuck to the floor while the rest of the body from the knee up is doing a pirouette, the medial collateral ligament has to suffer.

The fact that few injuries are incurred by the knee when it is in the air and not weight-bearing can be exploited by male dancers who are susceptible to knee problems. It follows that the shorter the length of time the foot is on the ground and weight-bearing, the less the likelihood of injuries. Thus, when lifting and traveling across the floor, a male dancer might possibly avert problems by making his steps more rapid and shorter.

HYPEREXTENSION

Strong supporting musculature is of particular importance

for the dancer with hyperextended or "swayback" knees. Any dancer with this problem should avoid exercises that over-stretch the hamstrings and contribute to joint laxity; for exam-ple, stretching with one leg extended and supported by only the ankle on the barre will only worsen the looseness behind the knee. Preferably, this type of stretch should be done with the leg supported above the knee, using a table top or a piano top instead of the barre. Dancers are often instructed to "pull up the thigh" or "pull up the hips"; since this actually involves locking of the knee, it can present a problem for the hyper-extended dancer, who will obviously end up "swaykneed" with tight locking. Compensation and straightening of the knees must therefore be achieved by a shifting of the weight forward by tilting the pelvis on the hip, while maintaining enough firm muscular control of the joint to hold it stable without locking.

KNEE PAIN

Pain around the kneecap can have various and sundry causes. Along the lower border it can result from excessive kneeling on hard floors, especially in male dancers who land solidly on one knee after a pirouette or tour en l'air. With continual friction and pressure, one of the bursa behind the knee frequently becomes irritated, a condition commonly known outside the dance world as "housemaid's knee" (in-flammation of a deeper bursa can be a much more serious problem). Buying kneepads for rehearsal is a good preventative investment, since an inflamed bursa can often make full exten-sion of the leg a real accomplishment. Another source of knee pain is excessive strain on the patellar ligament (part of the extensor apparatus of the leg, joining patella to tibia). So-called Jumper's Knee is by no means the sole domain of jumping dancers, as this vague but ubiquitous entity is known as High-

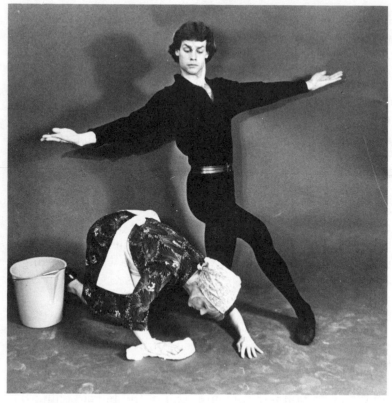

Housemaid's knee: a condition definitely not limited to housemaids. Photo by Dale Durfee

Jumper's Knee, Basketballer's Knee, Cross-Country Knee, Place-Kicker's Knee, and so on, depending on one's preference. Locking the knee with "pulling up" is another way to inflict excessive stretch to this region, as is working with knee hyperextension. And not surprisingly, "knee screwers" may also suffer knee pain, generally over the lower aspect as well.

CARTILAGE INJURY

The internal cartilage of the knee happens to be attached to the medial collateral ligament, which means that a severe sprain of the ligament can result in a meniscus tear or the cartilage's becoming a loose body in the joint. Loose cartilage can become caught in the articulating surfaces, resulting in joint locking. Even if properly replaced by manipulation, the cartilage will invariably continue to become displaced with successively less strain. A torn knee cartilage may not necessarily prevent a dancer from continuing work once the initial symptoms have settled, but sooner or later it will have to be surgically removed. Surgery of this type is usually well tolerated, with a cure possible in six to eight weeks. With proper rehabilitation, cartilage removal should not threaten a dancer's career.

SUBLUXED PATELLA

Occasionally a dancer will complain that her kneecap "goes out of place." This partial dislocation (or subluxation) of the patella is one of the few knee injuries that can occur while the knee is airborne and not weight-bearing. The mechanism appears to be an increased pull of the patella to the outside by the contracting quadriceps; it might occur, for example, during a series of piqué turns if the knee is not turned out and over the foot for the plié. For some reason, females are more susceptible to this problem; theories as to the cause include the increased angle of pull on the patella due to the wider hip structure of the female, poor quadriceps tone, and a congenitally shallow and flattened recess for the patella itself. Anytime the knee locks or gives out, immediate medical attention should be sought in order to rule out cartilage damage or patellar slippage.

CHONDROMALACIA

A condition which seems to be very prevalent in dancers (particularly those with a forced turn-out) is called chondromalacia patella, a softening of the knee cartilage. To some extent this condition is seen in almost all adults over thirty; it may be without symptoms in a large number of cases, but often it will manifest itself by pain behind the kneecap, stiffness after prolonged immobility, and pain with full extension. The initial site of the cartilage degeneration is nearly always the underside of the patella; although the exact cause is unknown, trauma to the area has been implicated, with the changes usually beginning at about age twenty. Treatment for the problem is variable and should be conservative unless disability and severity necessitate otherwise. Early degenerative change is an occupational hazard that a dancer will generally have no great difficulty in getting by with, but proper technique is probably as good a preventative measure as anything. Pain in the deep surface of the patella may be due to bruising or irritation of the cartilage and may be confused with the more permanent changes of chondromalacia—which again points out the good sense of having any pain properly evaluated by a physician. With knee involvement, conditions such as chondromalacia, bursitis, strain, and cartilage problems must be distinguished from one another.

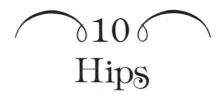

10
Hips

Turn-out is the foundation of all classical ballet. The ease with which it is obtained appears to correlate with the age at which dancing is begun and with consequent changes in ligaments. Most involved is the powerful, Y-shaped ilio-femoral ligament, which holds the head of the thighbone (femur) into the cup-shaped cavity (acetabulum) of the pelvis. It is part of the heavy network of ligamentous and fibrous tissue that forms a capsule enclosing the joint and (along with the strong supporting musculature and the deep socket) makes it the strongest joint in the body. Men generally begin training later than females and don't usually develop as extensive hip flexibility. General tightness around the hips has far-reaching ramifications; the back bears the brunt if called upon to compensate for a poor backward extension in arabesque; the foot, ankle, and knee suffer from improperly forcing a turn-out.

Six deep pairs of external rotators (obturator externus and internus, gemellus superior and inferior, quadrates femoris, and piriformis) and various accessory muscles (adductor magnus and brevis, gluteus maximus and medius, biceps femoris, iliopsoas, and sartorius) are the muscles responsible for turning out and maintaining turn-out, but the ligaments determine the possible range of motion. The degree of pure hip movement in a dancer's extension is a lot less than commonly realized. Normal movement at the joint involves only about sixty-five degrees forward, forty-five degrees to the side, and fifteen

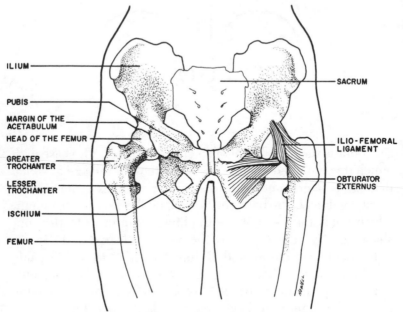

Hip and thigh anatomy (front view).

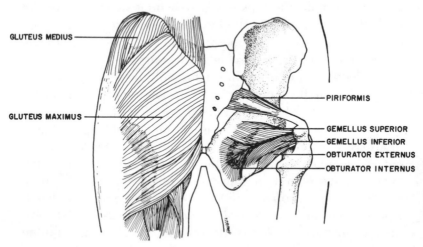

Hip and thigh anatomy (rear view).

degrees back (the ilio-femoral ligament prevents hyperextension more to the back than in any other direction). Beyond this
point, height is obtained by movement of the pelvis in relation
to the spine. This pelvic movement is greatly increased when
the body weight is on one leg—the pelvis rolls forward and
backward on the hipbone and twists or tilts from side to side. In
bending and rotation movements on one leg, it is practically
impossible to localize motion just to the spine itself.

The position of the pelvis in relation to the spine is as
important as its movement. The ligaments crossing the articulation between the last vertebrae of the spine (composing the
sacrum or tailbone) and the hip (consisting of the ischium,
ilium, and pubis bones fused together) are very strong; in fact,
it is debatable whether or not there is even enough leeway in
the joint for the "sacroiliac" sprain to really occur. Because of
this firm attachment the sacrum and hipbones move together
as one mass, the pelvis. Hence, "sticking the tailbone out"
causes an increase in the angle from which the lumbar spine
ascends upward from the sacrum, thereby increasing the hollow of the back. Similarly, the lumbar curve can be flattened
(with a corresponding flattening of the other curves) by "tucking in," tilting the pelvis in such a way that the takeoff of the
spine from the sacrum is more vertical. Thus, the normal
curvature of the back can be emphasized or decreased by pelvic
positioning; obviously, finding the correct centered placement
is essential for dance.

There are numerous bursae around the hip joint which, not
surprisingly, can become inflamed with overuse. The most
common sites of involvement are in front of the hip (pain
occurring with lifting the leg and turning inwards) and on the
outside of the thigh (pain particularly associated with movements à la seconde). As anywhere else, a flexible hip joint
without sufficient muscular strength and control is not advan-

tageous. A sudden twisting or turning can result in straining of muscles in the groin and on the inside of the upper thigh if they lack the tone to prevent overstretching (the latter, so-called rider's strain, is caused by too much stretch of the adductors when doing movements à la seconde). Some dancers with ligament laxity may even feel the thighbone "go out of joint"; this continual dislocating may lead to joint deterioration, so the importance of good muscle conditioning and avoidance of extreme stretching cannot be overemphasized. Always seek control more than height, and when warming up, don't risk strain by placing the leg on the barre for the first stretch.

11

Backs

A bad back and a good arabesque don't mix. Fortunately, serious disabling injuries of the back are unusual in a dancer who has a normal spine; unfortunately, since our spines are in the process of evolutionary change, a considerable amount of diversity (and error, even) accompanies the complex way in which backs are formed. Certain defects of the spine may go unnoticed until a dancer is challenged with a heavy schedule of lessons and rehearsals.

The spinal column is made up of a series of vertebrae, held together by muscles and ligaments and separated from each other by small pads of spongy elastic cartilage called intervertebral discs. The discs act as shock absorbers; they make up approximately one-fourth of the length of the spine and help to form the familiar natural curves by their variation in shape and thickness (a disc-less dancer would be about four feet tall and would have a slightly convex back from top to bottom). Although the back's curves aid in shock absorption, there is a slight weakening in the weight-bearing capacity as each curve merges into the next, especially in the low back region, where the backward curve of the thoracic vertebrae meets with the forward curve of the lumbar. Since all three curves (cervical, thoracic, and lumbar) must meet in the midline center of gravity to balance the weight distribution of the body, any alteration in one curve will affect the others; hence, a flat-backed person has decreased curvature throughout, while a hollow-backed person will have the compensating rounded shoulders and thorax.

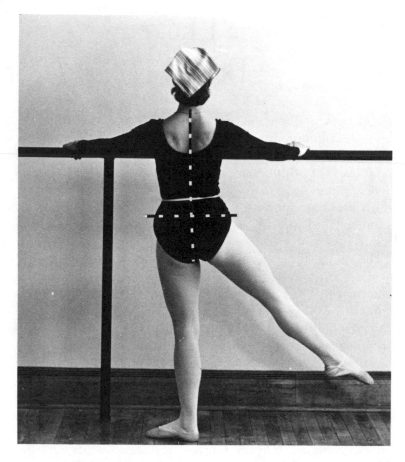

These two pictures attempt to demonstrate that pure hip movement is quite limited by the ilio-femoral ligament. With the leg only slightly lifted à la seconde (left), the axis of the pelvis is approximately perpendicular to that of the spine,

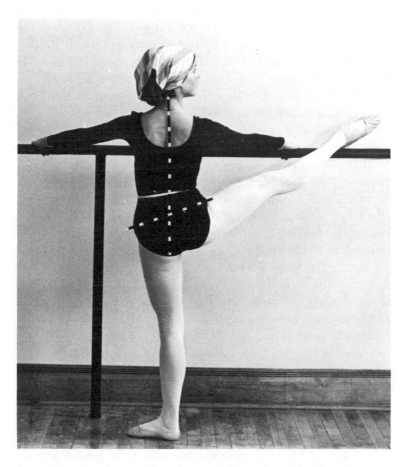

thus movement is predominantly of the femur in the hip
joint. Higher elevation of the leg (right) has been attained
by a considerable amount of tilting of the pelvis on the
spine.   Photos by Dale Durfee

Movement of the spinal column is in segments, with the vertebrae gliding and turning upon one another. The shapes of the individual bones as well as the manner in which they articulate to one another determine the range of motion. The first two vertebrae, for example (the atlas and axis), are specialized to allow free and unimpeded motion in the neck. Although backward bending occurs in the lumbar as well as the cervical region, it is very limited in the thorax, primarily because the protruding spinous processes impinge on one another with hyperextension (you will notice that even when gymnasts or contortionists perform pretzellike maneuvers, the upper torso moves more or less as one piece). Bending to the side takes place throughout the entire spine, but twisting is practically absent in the lumbar area. The degree of movement depends not only on the shape of the pieces and of the whole, but also on the length of the ligaments and the flexibility of the muscles—the latter being the main variable over which the dancer can exercise some control. Of course, movement of the back does not necessarily involve the spine alone; indirect movement is largely due to tilting of the pelvis, for example, and no amount of back flexibility is going to permit touching the palms to the ground with straight legs if the hamstrings are tight.

DISCS

Perhaps no medical term is used with more frequency and less understanding than "disc disease," probably because we have a desire to simplify into a single disease process a malady that doesn't seem to want to conform to a simplistic interpretation. The intervertebral discs take a lot of knocking about over the years, and they are subject to degeneration from the wear and tear. Undoubtedly, a person's particular constitution may

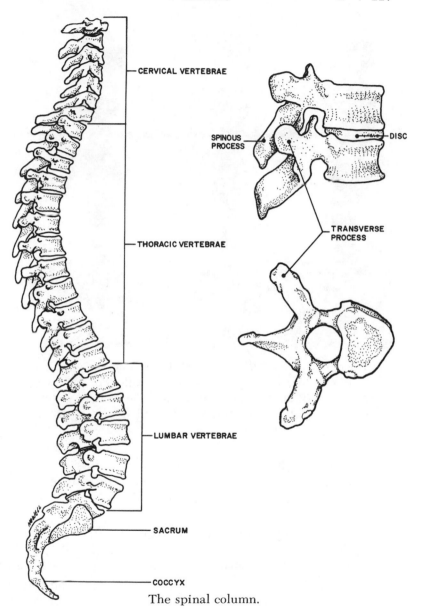

CERVICAL VERTEBRAE

SPINOUS PROCESS

DISC

THORACIC VERTEBRAE

TRANSVERSE PROCESS

LUMBAR VERTEBRAE

SACRUM

COCCYX

The spinal column.

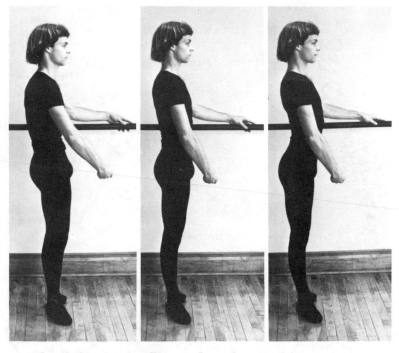

These photographs illustrate how the spinal curvature can be diminished by "tucking in" the pelvis (left) or increased by "sticking the tailbone out" (right). The middle picture shows correct centered placement, which isn't nearly as amusing.   Photos by Dale Durfee

predispose to earlier degeneration or vulnerability, as well as the amount of trauma or stresses that the body must endure. Posture, conditioning, and technique may come into play here for the dancer.

The disc in itself is insensitive to pain. Its upper and lower plates are the end plates of the adjacent vertebral bodies, made of inert articular hyaline cartilage. The wall of the disc, called the annulus, is an intertwining fibrous and elastic mesh that encapsulates the matrix (or nucleus pulposus), a gelatinous material that is about 80 percent water in a young, healthy spine. In this sense, the disc actually acts as an hydraulic type of shock absorber, the self-contained, noncompressible fluid accepting and transmitting the shock of compression forces. Supposing that because of disc degeneration, adjacent vertebral bodies come in closer approximation, allowing the supporting ligaments to bulge somewhat; or that due to increased stresses and activity, the supporting ligaments are stretched to allow some positional changes of the disc—in such instances pressure on the nearby nerve roots may result, and the pain will begin. In extreme cases, the gelatinous matrix material can even escape the confinement of its enveloping fibrous capsule and exert pressure—the so-called herniating or ruptured disc. Thus, by its action on surrounding structures, the intervertebral disc in some manner participates in the instigation of pain, a pain which is generally located in the low back and which often travels down one or both legs.

SPONDYLOLISTHESIS

Aside from the "slipped disc," there is a condition known as spondylolisthesis—far from a household word, but an important one for dancers, who have a higher incidence of this "true vertebral slipping" than the general population. Spondylolisthesis is usually the result of a slit in the posterior "arch" segment of a vertebral body, in the isthmus between the upper and lower articulations. This defect, called spondylolysis, is not permitted to heal because of continual movement of the spine. With loss of support (bony continuity may be completely broken with only the ligaments and muscles providing stability), the entire vertebral body and disc can slip forward on the vertebra below it. The severity of the resulting low back pain is not related to the extent of slippage; rather, it is related to the amount of muscle spasm resulting from the instability of the vertebra and to the impingement of the disc on the spinal nerves.

Spondylolysis is found in approximately 5 percent of the population, the vast majority of cases involving the fourth and fifth lumbar vertabrae, and is often completely asymptomatic throughout life. It is generally felt that the initiating bony defect is caused by numerous small stress fractures to the susceptible area, although certain people may be more vulnerable to the problem from birth (it is not strictly a congenital defect, however, since no instances have been found where the fracture was present from birth). The tendency for the fracture to progress to slippage is higher in dancers probably because of the continual stresses; the intensive early training may possibly be an important contributing factor.* Spondylolisthesis should theoretically be a contraindication for a dancer's acceptance into a school or company, but it does not necessarily mean the end of an established dancer's career, as the symptoms may abate with rest and proper conservative treatment. However, operative fusion of the joint may be a necessary treatment in severe cases.

STRAINS AND SUCH

Most dancers, fortunately, won't have to contend with disc disease and spondylolithesis, but they'll still have the chance to have problems with strains and, more seriously, sprains. Poor posture, bad placement, and attempting to exceed those basic

---

* In case anyone should ask, "What do ballet dancers, Welsh coal miners, and Eskimos have in common?" the answer is "an increased incidence of spondylolysis." In the latter two groups, postural stresses (be they from crouching in mines or huddling in igloos) are presumed to be the cause.

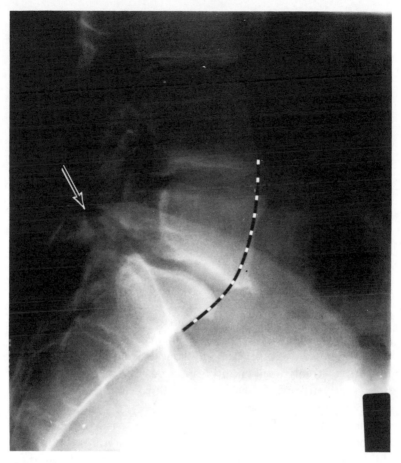

A fracture in the posterior arch of the fifth lumbar vertebra (arrow), or spondylolysis, has resulted in spondylolisthesis, slippage of the vertebral body forward on the vertebra below it (dashed lines indicate normal positioning).

anatomical limitations may all lead to back injury. The arabesque is the obvious culprit; strain can come about either with hyperextension of the back, or with failure to keep the pelvis level. Tightness around the hips can lead to lower back strain, particularly in male dancers; with limited extension at the hips, they may get into trouble by lifting the leg too high, then forcing the trunk upwards. Remember that a proper arabesque does not force all the movement at the bottom of the spine, but rather spreads the extension through all of the spinal joints. Male dancers will probably suffer more back strains than females because of the lifting they do, and they are especially vulnerable when fatigued or when the execution is improper.* In partnering, males should always avoid excess bending back in the lower back if they are positioned correctly; strengthening the arm and shoulder muscles, as well as correctly using the powerful leg extensors (when the lift starts with a plié), can minimize this occupational hazard.

Up along the spine about a foot or two, the neck is also particularly susceptible to strain because of the sudden whipping movement required for spotting turns and the fact that the neck is relatively weaker and in poorer condition than the less neglected parts of a dancer's body. Injuries in this area can also involve nerve pinch or stretch.

Back strains are for the most part treated as any other strain, the best treatment being rest (lying in the lateral position with the knees drawn up toward the abdomen is generally good for any acute low back pain). Heat or cold, specific exercises, massage, or ultrasound may be recommended by the physician; in more severe cases, a corset or plaster of Paris jacket

---

* The sex distribution of back strains and sprains from the workmen's compensation claims of a large professional ballet company substantiate my suspicions.

may be required for more adequate immobilization. Since the back has a more natural inclination for muscle spasm rather than strain, ice massage combined with a gradual stretch can often relieve some symptoms instantaneously. Remember, however, that "muscle spasm" is not a proper diagnosis for a back disorder, but is rather the back's natural response to various disorders or injuries.

Back pain is one of the most complex, if not frustrating, problems to deal with in medicine and, for the dancer, is certainly not a matter to trifle with. Any back pain that doesn't respond to a couple of days' rest with application of heat or cold is sufficient reason to contact an experienced physician. In particular, because of the tendency of dancers to develop spondylolysis and spondylolisthesis, all recurrent low back complaints should be thoroughly evaluated by a specialist. Finally, a word of caution concerning back manipulations: many dancers routinely employ chiropractors or others who practice these techniques. It is extremely important that dis-eased discs as well as spondylolisthesis not be manipulated; what is therapeutic in one instance can be disastrous in another. Most good chiropractors will take back films before doing any cracking—but play it safe; consult with your regular physician before going elsewhere for back manipulations. If he has experience with dancers, he may give you his blessing; in other instances, he may be very skeptical. Whatever his biases, if the practice is definitely contraindicated, his advice may keep you from incurring further injury and disability.

PART FOUR
Specific Generalities

12

Diet and Dieting

There is no love sincerer than the love of food.
—GEORGE BERNARD SHAW

Having trouble with turn-out? Eat shredded wheat for break-fast. Not pointing the feet? Egg rolls at the Imperial Palace (you'll have to come to Kansas City). And the secret's been out for years that salmon dip on Triscuits does wonders for extension.

Ludicrous? Not really much more farfetched than the food fallacies that have plagued mankind since his jaws began to work. Take the superstitions of primitive tribes: types of foods, in particular the meat of certain animals, endow the eater with the strength, speed, or whatever else happens to be the particular forte of the item ingested. Dare you to believe our misconceptions any more sophisticated, just talk to a football player in training who's chomping away on a rare cut of sirloin. The old "you-are-what-you-eat" diet.*

Dancers are especially prone to nutritional abuses because of the necessity of keeping weight down. Who in this world can have more of an obsession with diet than a 102-pound ballerina who disparagingly comments on her "three-and-a-half-pound obesity" as she refuses an extra teaspoon of wheat germ on her

---

* "Tell me what you eat, and I will tell you what you are," as Anthelme Brillat-Savarin (1755–1826) put it.

yogurt? The Greek Olympic athletes were also big ones on eating the proper foods—so much so, in fact, that Plato noted them "liable to most dangerous illnesses if they depart in ever so slight a degree from their customary regimen." Take it from the Greeks, there is absolutely no need for a rigidly defined pattern of eating—approximately fifty nutrients are recognized as essential to good health, and no single food comes close to containing even most of them. Diversity and flexibility are thus of major importance in any diet, as are self-control (if the scale tips more than it should) and common sense. Thanks to our knowledgeable body, many of us can get away with certain abuses; nonetheless, some dietary practices are as detrimental as they are foolish, particularly for a dancer who has to be at her peak. What follows is a brief touching upon a few facts and basic principles, a limited understanding of which might affect how and with what you fill your spoon.

CALORIES AND NUTRIENTS

The body daily consumes approximately 1,500 Calories* strictly for basic metabolic functions (about a third of this during sleep). In order to perform the most minimal necessary activities, add another 500, totaling 2,000 Calories for the average adult who remains in bed watching soap operas all day, leaving only to brush his teeth, use the toilet, and adjust the

---

* A calorie (lower case *c*) is defined as the amount of heat energy necessary to raise the temperature of a gram of water from 15 to 16 degrees centigrade, or, more practically, if you divide an Oreo into 50,000 equal pieces and eat one of them, you will have ingested 1 calorie. Since this is a fairly small amount, the unit of measurement commonly used is the Calorie (uppercase *C*), or kilocalorie (kcal), which is equal to 1,000 calories. From here on, I will only be referring to "big" calories, which is what nearly everybody takes for granted anyway.

fine tuning or volume controls (if this amount seems too great, keep in mind that this estimate is based on the "average" adult, who obviously weighs more—and hence has more tissue to maintain—than the "average" ballerina). For those who have to work or play, the amount of Calories consumed may vary from an additional 600 for a sedentary person to 3,000 for an active athlete. Using this information, along with the first law of thermodynamics (which goes something like "Matter is neither created nor destroyed, but rather converted from one form to another"), we can reason out the basic principle, which appears almost profound in its simplicity: namely, if energy consumption exceeds energy expenditure, weight will be gained, and if expenditure exceeds consumption, weight will be lost. Going logically one step further, the only two ways to lose weight are to increase energy expenditure or to decrease food intake. Just for some ballpark figures: since there are approximately 3,500 Calories stored in 0.5 kilogram (kg) of body fat (slightly more than one pound), this amount of energy must be expended in excess of intake for that amount of weight to be lost. In the other direction, a positive balance of approximately 2,500 Calories is required to provide for each 0.5 kg of increased weight of lean body tissue.* Considering that perhaps a ton of food, containing a million calories, will be consumed in the

---

* Don't let these concrete figures lull you into a false sense of security about calorie counting. Not only is precise measuring of energy intake and expenditure difficult, but estimates of energy changes in the body do not always conform to theoretical expectations. Thus, even if variables (such as amount of dancing, body size and composition, age, and dancing conditions) are similar, it is erroneous to assume that different individuals (or even the same individual at different times) will use food the same way or with the same efficiency. This should be no great revelation—doesn't everyone know some hateful dancer who seemingly can eat more without ever gaining an ounce?

span of a year, with probably little more than a few pounds' fluctuation, the weight-control process in most athletes is probably close to self-regulating.

But let's forget gaining and losing for a moment and consider our energy sources. Since a dancer obviously expends more energy than the average individual, she will require extra calories of intake just to stay in nutritional balance. The extra calories should be mainly in the form of carbohydrate, the most efficient fuel for muscle and the foodstuff used almost exclusively during heavy physical exertion and endurance events. Excess carbohydrate is stored in liver and muscle in the form of glycogen. When these stores are decreased with prolonged physical activity, fatigue ensues, generally reflecting low blood sugar levels. Symptoms may include weakness, headache, irritability, nervousness, and a loss of mechanical efficiency due to faulty coordination. Since the best time to replenish the glycogen stores is two to three days prior to a performance, it makes absolutely no sense for a dancer to cut back on carbohydrate shortly before a performance for the sake of a pound or two.

On the other hand, some athletes, particularly long-distance runners, go overboard by a practice called carbohydrate loading. Vigorous exercise while on a low carbohydrate diet followed by light exercise and high carbohydrate intake can cause the glycogen content of muscle to more than double, thus increasing endurance. This is the only nutritional manipulation known to increase athletic performance, but it is not advisable. Associated with this routine is a tremendous increase in water deposition with the risk of stiffness and heaviness, chest pain and electrocardiogram changes, and the possible destruction of muscle fibers.

Fats are used by the body as a fuel for low intensity exercise and are not as efficient an energy source as carbohydrate. Since

fat is more dense calorically than either carbohydrate or protein (about 9 Calories per gram for fat and about 4 Calories per
gram for both carbohydrate and protein), it is easier to take
extra calories, if desired, as fat. By the same token, increasing
the percentage of fat in the diet is the surest way to pick up
added baggage. A desirable amount of fat in the diet is in the
range of 30–35 percent of total caloric intake, certainly no more
than 45 percent. Some fats are necessary in a well-balanced
diet because of vitamins and certain essential fatty acids contained in them, as well as what appears to be a fat-contained
substance that is needed for normal carbohydrate metabolism.

Protein (from the Greek, meaning literally "to take first
place") is a molecule composed of smaller segments called
amino acids. There are twenty-two different amino acids, and
all but eight—the essential amino acids—can be synthesized
by the body. An adequate intake of protein in the adult diet is
about 11 or 12 percent of the total calories, and athletes require
no more than less active individuals. Protein contributes to the
growth and maintenance of human tissue but is not an efficient
energy fuel. Any excess of the daily requirement is either
excreted through the kidneys or converted into fat and stored.
For some reason, we don't think of meat as ending up as stored
fat—perhaps a holdover from our ancient food myths. But
muscle mass does not increase in proportion to the mass of
ingested protein; it increases only through muscle work. So
eating more food—even as protein—will only add fat unless
accompanied by exercise and training.

VITAMINS

Vitamins are necessary for the normal metabolic functioning
of the body but do not provide energy or build tissues in
themselves. Dancing does not increase vitamin or mineral

requirements. Reasonable vitamin supplementation may be helpful (and certainly can't do any harm), but, unfortunately, many dancers view vitamins as a cure-all or a replacement for a proper diet. Actually, the converse is true. Any balanced diverse diet (with a selection of foods from each of the four larger groups: milk, meat, vegetable/fruit, and bread/cereal) will generally supply all the needed amounts of vitamins. Since the percentage of dancers eating well-balanced diets is probably not staggering, this may very well be a moot point.

Certain vitamins in particular are enjoying the notoriety implicit in the typically American "more-is-better" philosophy. There is absolutely no scientific support for claims that megadoses of vitamins are beneficial. Some vitamins are toxic and may be life-threatening in larger doses, particularly Vitamins A, D, and K. The approximately 4,000 cases of vitamin poisoning reported each year by the Food and Drug Administration are good testimony against the commonly held notion of the harmlessness of vitamins. Megadoses of Vitamin E have not been shown to lengthen life, enhance sexual powers, clear up blemishes, or accomplish any of the other numerous claims. Nor have megadoses of Vitamin C been shown to cure the common cold; in fact, some researchers are trying to prove that large doses of C actually increase the body's destruction of it, leaving the taker relatively deficient upon discontinuance of massive supplementation. Niacin supplementation is definitely contraindicated for the dancer, since niacin has been found to inhibit the heart muscle's uptake of fatty acids during exercise. On the other hand, appropriate iron supplementation for the ballerina is probably advisable, since an estimated 15–20 percent of all female athletes are relatively iron deficient.

SHEDDING POUNDS

As mentioned previously, weight can be lost either by increasing energy expenditure or decreasing caloric intake. For the active dancer, the advice "get more exercise" isn't very helpful (although it's probably the major factor involved in weight gain for the injured dancer who can't maintain her regular training schedule). Which leaves us with cutting back on calories, which no one wants to hear. But if you have faith in the first law of thermodynamics, there's no surer way and no shortcut.

The most crucial thing about a weight-reduction program is that the diet contain optimal intake of all the essential nutrients—a dieter should not have to depend on vitamin, mineral, or protein supplements any more than any other healthy individual. Oddball and fad diets usually make overblown claims and are often nutritionally unsound. The best bet is to feast on an adequate mixed diet, while cutting down on helpings. If fatty foods are too large a percentage of daily intake, selectively cutting back more on fats will be helpful. A dieter must set his or her own priorities and make choices; if a person can absolutely not survive without a Hostess Twinkie every day, then 185 or so odd calories will have to be eliminated somewhere else. Which reminds me—"good" food (like Twinkies) is not necessarily bad provided it is a part of an overall well-balanced diet.* In any event, total caloric intake

---

* Junk foods are given a bad name not from an energy standpoint, but rather because increasing consumption of sucrose has been incriminated in the causation of coronary artery disease, obesity, and diabetes, among others. Due to modern technology, the change of carbohydrate sources from starch (derived principally from cereals and potatoes) to purified sugars (sucrose from sugar cane or sugar beet, and glucose-fructose mixtures from cornstarch) has been considerable. Purified sugars now contribute an estimated 15–25 percent of the total caloric intake of Americans (a moderate 5–10 percent would probably be a better range).

should never be less than 2,000 Calories per day for a working dancer, and weight loss should be given a significant time period—about a couple of pounds a week is usually the desired rate, and it should probably never be double that amount. All things being equal, reducing caloric intake by 500 Calories per day or 3,500 Calories per week is theoretically the energy equivalent of 0.5 kg body fat.

Put in those terms, it sounds pretty easy, but if it were, there wouldn't be so many overweight people running around in this country (about one in five adults). The problem with dancers who have diet hassles does not seem to be a lack of will power so much as impatience and a tendency to procrastinate. A dancer will go for weeks with five pounds extra on board (complaining nonstop), and then will proceed to demonstrate her self-control by starving herself the week before the season's opening. Aside from depletion of glycogen stores, rapid weight losses are not compatible with either maintenance of muscle mass or satisfactory performance, the reason being that diets change body composition as well as reducing weight. When the body's fat and glycogen stores are reduced (and dancers obviously have less surplus fat than nontrained persons), needed calories will be drawn from breakdown of body protein. A semistarvation diet (especially with water and salt deprivation) results in weight loss in the form of protein, glycogen, potassium, phosphorus, sodium, and other minerals and trace elements—at least half of the weight loss being fat-free. So we have a dizzy, nauseated, dehydrated, and fatigued dancer. But at least she can't complain about being overweight.

Rapid weight fluctuations—a couple of pounds or more in a 24-hour period—are due to fluid shifts and do not represent fat loss or gain. Approximately 65 percent of a male's body weight is water, with the specific percentage depending upon the individual's ratio of fat to muscle (fat contains only about 20 percent water, while muscle contains a whopping 75 percent). It is of the utmost importance to maintain a good state of hydration by adequate intake of salt and water, particularly in warm, humid studios and in periods of heat acclimation. Dehydration compromises energy metabolism and limits endurance, and can be life threatening if extreme. Obviously, water pills (diuretics) for weight loss only compound the dehydration, potassium loss, and muscle weakness, and should never be used. Nor are other pills, such as stimulants, ever indicated in the dancer either for purposes of stifling appetite or combating fatigue.

Another misconception and possible abuse is the use of rubber or plastic suits. These garments produce only fluid loss, not true fat weight loss, and possibly can precipitate heat stroke. Don't be led to believe that you can selectively trim down those thighs; even though some of those products are deceptively marketed as "slimming," observe that the accompanying literature rightly seems more concerned with precautions than with the alleged weight-reducing properties. If you insist on wearing them, wear them as warmers (they're cheaper than knit warmers, anyway), and wear them judiciously. They definitely do insulate well, and are fine for keeping the muscles warm backstage. However, if used continuously in a warm studio, they function less as warmers than as "dehydrants."

PREPERFORMANCE EATS

Probably everyone knows at least one dancer who snarfs down a greasy double-burger, onion rings, and a strawberry milkshake, dabs her lips demurely with a napkin, and immediately proceeds to make a leaping entrance onstage. For the vast majority of us, though, with relatively normal gastrointestinal tracts, there are certain guidelines for preperformance meals.

After food is eaten, a relatively greater amount of blood is shunted through the vessels of the digestive system to aid in digestion, leaving a proportionally smaller amount to supply muscles during strenuous exercise. If the circulation to the muscles falls off, cramping may result (swimmer's cramp is the perfect example). On the other hand, if more of the blood goes to the muscles in preference to fulfilling the commitment to the gut, indigestion and poor food absorption may be the result, which can sometimes lead to diarrhea and/or vomiting. Ideally, a good-sized meal should be eaten at least two hours, but preferably more, before performing, since it usually takes two hours for food to travel through the stomach, and another two for it to pass through the small intestine. The preferred type of food is bland, nongreasy, and easily digestible, with a relatively high carbohydrate content. Generally to be avoided are large amounts of protein (which stimulate acid secretion in the stomach), fat (which delays digestion), and gas-producing foods such as beans, cucumbers, and radishes.

⌒ ♦13 ♦ ⌒

Medical Care
and Rehabilitation

How poor are they that have not patience!
What wound did ever heal but by degrees?
—IAGO

Dancers are hypercritical of the slightest abnormality, yet often hesitant to seek attention for physical problems. The denial of possible injury may come from the fear that dancing will have to be cut back or cease—that something really is the matter. Or the fear may be directed toward a demanding choreographer. And finally, the old philosophy of "being a trooper" still pervades. Nonetheless, the problems of appropriate health care don't end with consulting a specialist for evaluation, they just begin. Whether or not a dancer is stubborn and impatient, most assuredly he or she will be action-oriented. Hippocrates stated that sometimes "the best treatment is to do nothing," and while this may often be true, the "no-treatment treatment" is very difficult for the dancer's psyche.

The choreography of healing is basically Mother Nature's; medications and physical therapy modalities cannot really alter the normal healing process. For example, connective fibrous tissue heals by the formation of a mature scar in approximately four to six weeks. If the injury to a ligament is incomplete or

137

minor, perhaps a healing period of only three to four weeks will be sufficient. Appropriate medical care can minimize the initial tissue reaction (bleeding into the tissues and swelling), prevent further damage to vulnerable surrounding areas (proper stabilization of the damaged area), facilitate healing (alleviating spasm and pain, providing an appropriate environment for healing by various physical therapy modalities), and prevent excessive fibrous thickening in the area (gradual exercise rehabilitation). But there is more to deal with than just the isolated site of injury. Equally important is the maintenance of overall body conditioning (keeping the uninjured parts and the heart and lungs in shape), keeping weight down, and making sure that the sidelined dancer does more than brood or climb the walls.

Although certain types of injuries may necessitate almost total immobilization, these are the exception rather than the rule, and most physicians will try hard to prevent the cure being worse than the disease. Treatment should ideally be directed toward that which will do no harm while helping to keep the rest of the body (and mind) fit. An important consideration is the extent of muscle atrophy with disuse—for every week of rest, a similar period of training is estimated to be required to bring the body back to the preinjury conditioning level. The vast majority of dance problems may be successfully treated with modification rather than limitation of activity; for example, avoiding jumps or full pliés, doing restricted barre work only, or establishing a specific rehabilitative exercise program. Often it is a good idea for injured dancers to use the swimming pool; muscles can be stretched out, weight can be worked off, and barre work may be possible, using the buoyancy of the water to diminish the weight and strain on a recovering working leg.

Physicians experienced in working with dancers have a very

pragmatic attitude. They will be fairly open-minded concerning ancillary personnel, and may refer patients to massage therapists, acupuncturists, or special gymnasiums. They understand the tendency of dancers to be faddists and are generally more willing to cater to, or at least indulge them in, their psychological needs. What is of concern is the health of the dancer in the broadest sense, and anything that brings relief, be it psychological or otherwise, without having physically harmful ramifications, should probably be tolerated. There is a big difference between a qualified acupuncturist who may be able to relieve pain (with the understanding that this relief does nothing to remedy the underlying cause) and a quack who claims he can "realign and straighten everything in two weeks and for only $1,500." It is unfortunate that a lack of empathy on the part of a physician can sometimes precipitate a visit to a manipulator who can do more harm than good.

Competent physicians may have differing approaches to the same type of problems because of their particular experience and therapeutic biases. Some prefer cold to heat in the healing stages; some swear by deep heat, while others feel superficial to be adequate; some use drugs and others don't. Probably all get equally good results, mainly because the body is running most of the show by itself, with the help of rest and time. Perhaps a good number of the therapies are more psychologically palliative as "mental sedatives" than anything else; but if the Saran Wrap or soaks or balms feel like they're doing good, then in one way or another they probably are.

Not everybody dances in New York, Boston, or Los Angeles, and it may be somewhat of a chore to find a physician who deals with a lot of dancers if you happen to live in Dismal Seepage, Kansas. Even in larger communities, the resources for certain physical therapy modalities may not be as readily available or as financially feasible as they might be for a large company that provides insurance coverage and a company physician. How do you select a specialist? The best advice is to seek a referral from your family physician, try to get an appointment with a team physician (if there is one), or else go to the biggest jock you can find (my first choice for an orthopedist was a former Michigan football player, and it was a good one). If the best you can do is a family physician who only treats an occasional "weekend warrior" (the kind that says "you'll be all right if you lay off of it for a couple of months"), take the initiative by inquiring more specifically as to the extent of the injury and limitations, then ask if he has any suggestions for permissible forms of activity. If he has none, suggest your own (flat-footed barre, swimming, physical therapy), and in most instances you will jointly come up with something, no matter how little he knows about dancing and dancers (at least he, one hopes, knows about medicine; you can remedy his deficiencies).

A brief word at this point on drugs. Local pain from an injury can usually be best controlled by immobilization and cold, and in most medically minor injuries, little more than a mild analgesic is needed, if anything is needed at all. The use of painkillers masks symptoms, often delaying proper care at the proper time and destroying guidelines for logical control of rehabilitation. Because it destroys pain sensitivity and produces local swelling, injection of local anaesthetics or steroids (with a few specific exceptions) is a condemned practice. Many physicians routinely prescribe muscle relaxants or antiinflammatory agents; the possible benefits must be balanced against possible undesirable side effects, particularly stomach upsets. As with any drug, they should only be taken upon the advice or prescription of a physician. Nothing contains more truth than the old saying, "He who treats himself has a fool for a doctor," particularly where medications are concerned.

The best medicine is always preventative. Any cure will only be temporary if there is some underlying cause determining the reason for injury. A bad habit, technical inadequacy, or improper dance conditions can be changed. A defect in anatomy can be a bit harder to deal with, but even in these cases there may sometimes be methods of compensation, surgical or otherwise. We continue to learn more about the body, in some cases only to prove or explain something that dancers have known for years. The potential for feeding back new knowledge and understanding into ballet training and health care for the dancer is great and most exciting. Yet that which the dancer gives—that ethereal spark of magic—will always be beyond the vision and comprehension of any dissection.

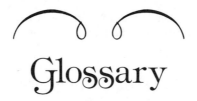

Glossary

ABDUCTION. The movement of a body part away from the midline.

ACETABULUM. The cup-shaped cavity of the hip bone in which the head of the femur fits.

ACUTE. Pertaining to an injury, of sharp and sudden onset.

ADDUCTION. The movement of a body part toward the midline.

ADHESIONS. Fibrous bands adhering parts to one another (particularly in relationship to the opposing surfaces of a wound).

ALUM. A crystalline substance used as an astringent.

ANTAGONIST. A muscle working in opposition to the action of another muscle.

ARTICULATION. A joint.

ASTRINGENT. A substance that causes contraction of the tissues and arrests secretions and bleeding.

ATROPHY. A wasting away of tissues.

AVULSION. The tearing away of a part from the whole.

BALLISTIC STRETCH. Stretching obtained by bouncing, bobbing, or lunging.

BENZOIN (TINCTURE OF). A gum-resin derivative used for its mild antiseptic and protectant effects, especially prior to the application of adhesive tape.

BLISTER. A collection of fluid under or within the skin layers.

BUNION. An inflamed, thick-walled bursa over the first metatarsophalangeal joint, usually associated with the hallux valgus deformity.

BUROWS SOLUTION. Aluminum acetate solution used as a foot soak by some dancers.

BURSA. A closed, fluid-filled sac usually found or formed in areas subjected to friction.

BURSITIS. Inflammation of a bursa.

CALCANEUS Heel bone.

CALLUS A thickening of the skin as a result of friction or pressure.

CALORIE A unit of heat. The small calorie is the amount of heat required to raise the temperature of one gram of water from 15 degrees to 16 degrees centigrade. The large calorie (or kilocalorie) is the amount of heat required to raise the temperature of 1,000 grams of water from 15 degrees to 16 degrees centigrade.

CARTILAGE A specialized fibrous connective tissue. The hyaline variety is a bluish-white surface covering over certain bony articulations that absorbs shock, prevents direct wear on bones, and alters the fit of the joint.

CHARLEYHORSE. Technically, a contusion of the quadriceps; more commonly, muscle cramping, particularly of the lower leg.

CHIROPRACTOR. A practitioner of chiropractic, the system of therapeutics that attributes disease processes to malalignment of the vertebrae and hence treats disease by manipulation of the spinal column.

CHONDROMALACIA. Softening of cartilage.

CHRONIC. Persisting over a long period of time; not acute.

CONTRAST BATH. The therapeutic use of alternating hot and cold soaks.

CONTUSION. Bruise.

CORN. A localized callus caused by pressure over a bony prominence, usually a toe.

CRAMP. A painful muscular contraction or spasm.

DANCER'S HEEL. A common term for pain above the heel bone in the Achilles area, presumedly caused by joint inflammation secondary to trauma.

DEHYDRATION Reduction of water content from the body.

DIARTHRODIAL JOINT. A bony articulation in which the opposing surfaces are covered with hyaline cartilage, there is a joint cavity containing synovial fluid and reinforced by a fibrous capsule, and free movement is more or less possible.

DIATHERMY. Deep heating of the tissues achieved by various forms of penetrating physical energy.

DISC (INTERVERTEBRAL). A pad of cartilage interposed between the bodies of adjacent vertebrae.

DORSIFLEXION. Bending of the foot upwards.

EVERSION.Lifting the outer border of the foot, or "rolling."

EXTENSION. The straightening of a body part or returning from flexion.

FASCIA A sheet of fibrous tissue that encloses and separates muscle.

FEMUR.The long bone of the thigh.

FIXATOR. A muscle which contracts isometrically to stabilize the origin of the prime mover so it can work efficiently.

FLEXION.A bending or folding movement in which the angle between the bone surfaces decreases.

FRACTURE.The breaking of continuity of a bone.

HALLUX RIGIDUS. Bony degenerative disease of the metatarsophalangeal joint of the great toe.

HALLUX VALGUS. A deviation of the tip of the great toe toward the outside (lateral aspect) of the foot.

HAMMER TOE.Deformity in which the first toe bone points upwards, while the second and third phalanges are flexed downwards.

HAMSTRING GROUP The muscles at the back of the thigh involved with thigh extension and knee flexion (biceps femoris, semitendinosus, semimembranosus).

HEMARTHROSIS Bleeding into a joint.

HEMATOMA A confined, localized mass of extravasated blood.

HEMOGLOBIN. The oxygen-carrying component of red blood cells.

HEMORRHAGE. Bleeding.

HOT SPOT. A reddened area of skin from friction.

HOUSEMAID'S KNEE. A painful knee condition resulting from inflammation of the prepatellar bursa.

HYPEREXTENSION. Extreme extension of a limb or part; for example, sway-back knees.

HYPERTROPHY. The enlargement of a body part due to an increase in cell size.

INFLAMMATION. The response of tissues to injury, with the classical signs of heat, pain, redness, and swelling.

INVERSION. Raising the inner border of the foot.

ISOMETRIC CONTRACTION. Contraction of muscle accompanied by increase in tension without change in length.

ISOTONIC CONTRACTION. Contraction of muscle accompanied by shortening in length.

JUMPER'S KNEE Knee pain caused by excessive strain of the patellar ligament.

KINESIOLOGY. The study of movement.

LATERAL. Pertaining to a position farther from the midline of the body or structure (as opposed to the medial or inner side).

MACERATION. Softening by the action of liquid.

MALLEOLUS.One of the bony protuberances on either side of the ankle joint.

MARCH FRACTURE.A stress or fatigue fracture involving a metatarsal bone.

MASSAGE.Therapeutic stroking of the body.

MEDIAL.Closer to the midline of the body or a structure (as opposed to the lateral or outer side).

MENISCUS.A crescent-shaped cartilage in the knee joint (medial and lateral).

METABOLISM.The sum total of all chemical and physical processes—constructive as well as destructive—by which the human organism is maintained.

MICROWAVE.The variety of diathermy utilizing energy in the form of electromagnetic waves.

MYOTATIC REFLEX. Reflex contraction of a muscle in response to excessive stretch.

ORTHOPEDIST. A physician specializing in the skeletal system, its articulations, and associated structures.

OS TRIGONUM. A small bone which may be either separate from or fused to the rear part of the talus.

OSTEOPATH. A practitioner of the school of medicine that employs manipulative measures in addition to the diagnostic and therapeutic measures of ordinary medicine.

OSTEOPOROSIS.Reduction in quantity of bone; bony atrophy.

PATELLA. Kneecap.

PHYSIOTHERAPY (PHYSICAL THERAPY). The use of physical agents such as light, heat, air, water, massage, exercise, or mechanical apparatus in the treatment of disease.

PLANTAR FLEXION. Bending the foot downwards.

PODIATRIST An individual who treats foot disorders.

PRIME MOVER. The chief muscle or chief member of a muscle group responsible for a particular movement.

PRONATION. Of the foot, a combination of abduction and eversion, resulting in a lowering of the medial edge of the foot.

QUADRICEPS GROUP. The muscles at the front of the thigh involved with thigh flexion and knee extension (rectus femoris, vastus lateralis, vastus intermedius, vastus medialis).

ROLLING. Improper weight distribution in which the medial border of the foot bulges inwards (eversion).

ROTATION. The pivoting of a bone on its axis (internal—toward the body midline; external—away from the body midline).

RUBEFACIENT An agent that produces reddening of the skin when applied topically.

SCREWING THE KNEE. A technical flaw in which turn-out is obtained by rotation of the tibia on the femur instead of from the hip.

SHIN SPLINTS. Pain and discomfort in the middle of the leg usually associated with excessive use of the foot flexors.

SHORTWAVE. The variety of diathermy utilizing high frequency electric current.

SICKLING. The rolling inward or outward of the foot and ankle while on demi-pointe.

SPASM. Sudden, involuntary contraction of a muscle or muscle group.

SPONDYLOLISTHESIS. Forward displacement of a vertebra on the one below it.

SPONDYLOLYSIS. A break in bony continuity of a vertebra.

SPRAIN. Tearing of ligament fibers.

SPUR. A projecting piece of bone.

STEROIDS. A large group of chemical substances (including hormones, vitamins, body constituents, and drugs), some of which are utilized for their antiinflammatory qualities.

STONE BRUISE. Contusion on the bottom of the foot, usually the result of repeated pounding on a hard surface or stepping on a small hard object.

STRAIN. Tearing of muscle fibers anywhere along a muscle or tendon (synonomous with "pull").

STRESS FRACTURE (FATIGUE FRACTURE). A fracture occurring as a consequence of accumulated impact and shock without any relationship to a single specific traumatic incident.

SUBLUXATION. An incomplete or partial dislocation.

SUPINATION. Of the foot, a combination of adduction and inversion, resulting in the raising of the inner edge of the foot.

SYNERGIST. A muscle that aids in the general movement or stabilizes intermediate joints to prevent unwanted movements.

SYNOVIA (SYNOVIAL FLUID). The viscous fluid resembling egg white which acts as a lubricant in joint cavities, bursae, and tendon sheaths.

TAILOR'S BUNION. A bunion on the outside of the fifth toe.

TALUS. Ankle bone.

TENDON. A fibrous cord attaching muscle to bone.

TENDINITIS. Inflammation of a tendon.

ULTRASOUND. The variety of diathermy utilizing mechanical vibrations as the penetrating source of energy.

UNGUIS INCARNATUS. Ingrown toenail.